Think Again!

Think Again!

*Clearing Away the
Brain Fog of Menopause*

JEANNE D. ANDRUS,
THE MENOPAUSE GURU

NEW YORK

NASHVILLE • MELBOURNE • VANCOUVER

Think Again!
Clearing Away the Brain Fog of Menopause

© 2018 **JEANNE D. ANDRUS**

Published in New York, New York, by Morgan James Publishing in partnership with Difference Press. Morgan James is a trademark of Morgan James, LLC. www.MorganJamesPublishing.com

The Morgan James Speakers Group can bring authors to your live event. For more information or to book an event visit The Morgan James Speakers Group at www.TheMorganJamesSpeakersGroup.com.

ISBN 978-1-68350-619-5 paperback
ISBN 978-1-68350-620-1 eBook
Library of Congress Control Number: 2017909091

Cover Design by:
Chris Treccani
www.3dogdesign.net

Interior Design by:
Bonnie Bushman
The Whole Caboodle Graphic Design

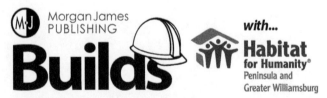

In an effort to support local communities, raise awareness and funds, Morgan James Publishing donates a percentage of all book sales for the life of each book to Habitat for Humanity Peninsula and Greater Williamsburg.

Get involved today! Visit
www.MorganJamesBuilds.com

To Hillary, Elizabeth, and Michelle,
because you have given much and I owe you much.

Table of Contents

Introduction

Let's talk about menopause and how it changes women. Especially how it changes their thinking. In fact, let's get personal. Let me tell you about how it changed me—about my experience with brain fog and the other ways menopause seems to attack our brains.

I used to be one of "those people"—you know them. They never need a list, they never forget a name, they always know where to look for their car keys, not because they always put them in the same place, but because they remembered they put them in the refrigerator. I can't believe I'm admitting that I was such an annoying type of person. Just kidding, of course, and if you were one of those people, you know exactly what I mean. It's hard to believe now that that was me.

When the changes of menopause, the ones that happened to my brain, happened to me, I freaked out. Frequently. Partly because I forgot things—big things, little things, any things. Partly because I found myself constantly starting over or going to turn in a report or a project only to realize that I'd only written half of the most important paragraph. And partly because I just didn't feel sharp, present, or smart anymore. I felt like my brain was wrapped in cotton candy, and it didn't even taste very good.

Oh, when I was younger, there were hints of it. I sometimes got a bad case of "walked through a door and forgot why I'm here." I had my own special version of that. My brain had two separate calendars: work things and not work things. It was easy to double book myself if there was a "work thing" and a "not work thing" happening at the same time. I did that when my son was in high school and I'd invariably schedule a late afternoon meeting on the day of his big cross-country meet. But, back then, I thought of those as my "adorable little foibles," and didn't give them a second thought.

So, when it seemed like my brain stopped working, that's when I got scared! Sure, the weight gain of perimenopause was annoying. And I wasn't wild about the wrinkles and gray hair (especially the way my gray was coming in). And, no, I didn't like that my periods weren't predictable. But when it came to my brain? Well, that was a different matter. That's when things got serious. Things got really serious.

If you're reading this book, I expect it's because you'd like to understand what's happening to you and your brain as you go through the process of menopause. Or maybe just what *might* happen to you. Even more importantly, you'd like to fix it. You'd like to *think* again. To have the fog lift. To be able to concentrate. To stop feeling like you're more distractible than a four-year-old boy at Disney World.

What this book is all about is what's going on in your brain (and the science behind it) and what you can do about it—because menopause doesn't have to be misery. I'll even help you find the magic.

Let's get started.

Chapter One

The Gift of Fog

—•—

Several years ago, when I started exploring the topic that just kept coming up for me—menopause—I realized that there were gifts and wisdom in many of the symptoms we experience. In each of my books, I have tried to explore the message, the wisdom, of the changes that occur, the symptoms that annoy us. These messages are often personal and, by listening to them, you can determine why you, in particular, might experience a specific symptom as more annoying or pervasive or intrusive.

I've tried to make it clear that I consider menopause to be a true gift to women, one that allows us to turn back into our deepest core and examine the life we've lived to date and decide what more we want to draw into our lives and experience now that we are older.

But, it hasn't always been easy seeing the gift in some of the more annoying symptoms. As for brain fog and the memory and thinking issues we're exploring here? This is probably the hardest one for me to find the gift in. It's hard for me to even consider that there might be a "silver lining" to brain fog—much less a gem of untold worth in it—because we're talking about my (and your) beautiful brains here! The ones that have gotten us this far, with whatever grace and elegance and brilliance they've had. They're the ones that hold the pictures of our babies, that took us through school, that communicate and direct and control. If my brain is on the fritz, I'm in big trouble. Aren't you?

I'm going take you with me on the journey I experienced as I prepared to write this chapter, because, even though I'd committed to telling you what the gift of brain fog is, I had no idea myself what it was.

Until this week, when the lock magically opened itself for me.

The Walk

Like many of you, I am inordinately proud of my kid (I only have one; if I had more, I'd be proud of them, too). And I am incredibly in love with my grandson, who just turned one year old as I have been writing this book. I lament daily the reality of the 1,800 miles or so that separate our homes and that mean I see my son and my grandson so rarely. So, when a business trip took me close enough to where they live for me to detour to join in the festivities for my grandson's first birthday, I jumped at the opportunity.

Saturday, of course, was filled with watching a child smash his first birthday cake into his high chair tray, his clothes, and his hair. My ex was there, so I also got caught up with the superficialities of his life and let him have a glimpse into mine. I admired my son's equanimity with the chaos in his life and delighted in getting to know the new person in my life—my grandson—on a whole new level.

Then came Sunday. My daughter-in-law was off to run a half-marathon, and I was delighted to have my son and grandson to myself for the day. (Hey, nothing against her, but what mom doesn't get excited for a date with the two most captivating men she knows?)

A drizzly, late fall day in northern New England may not be what everyone considers perfect hiking weather, but my son assured me that there was nothing his little guy liked more than a ride on his daddy's back through the woods. So we bundled up and headed out to one of their favorite trails. As the access road wound up the mountain, I watched the drizzle on the windshield turn to spitting snow and felt my own delighted anticipation. New Orleans, my home, might have lots of things, but opportunities for going hiking in weather like that isn't among them.

As we pulled in to a parking area, my son explained his trail choice. "It's funny," he said. "People think I'm nuts for preferring weather like this and for choosing trails that don't have the big vistas, the great views. But, really, being out here today, in this foggy weather, encourages me to look at all the small things, to examine what I see right here in front of me."

For the next two hours, we looked. We saw. We examined. We communed and reconnected with each other, with ourselves, and with the earth. We never reached a "scenic overlook" and, even if we had, there'd have been nothing to see but clouds. We never saw the other mountains surrounding us or even had a sense that there was anything beyond the small section of trail we covered. But there was a richness in what we did see and feel and experience and that brings a taste and a smell to my mind from just the act of describing it here.

The sky didn't part, a rainbow didn't appear, the sword didn't rise from the water. And yet, I felt, in those moments, during that hike, the clicking of the first tumbler of that lock. *22 Right.*

The Circle

Two days later, I left for my business meeting. But the business meeting was more than only business. It was a mastermind get-together, a trust circle, and a prayer meeting, too. It was a house party and a reunion and a gathering of the sisterhood in utmost solemnity and hilarity. What happened for most of the week is not mine to tell. But this next part I'm going to tell you is.

We gathered in a circle to celebrate not one, but the three birthdays among us that occurred during our time together. It was a joyous celebration of three amazing colleagues that turned even more special as we reflected on the special qualities each of us, not just our "birthday girls," brought to our collaborations. As I took my place in the center of the circle, I reflected on being the focus of everyone's attention as my qualities, strengths, and persona were reflected back to me through the mirror of my peers. I was being made aware of what they saw in me, and of being forced to acknowledge those things in myself.

Now, you might be scratching your head a little here. That was supposed to be all positive stuff they were telling me, right? What could be so difficult about hearing all kinds of wonderful stuff about yourself? Why would that be daunting or intimidating or scary? Let me assure you that when the circle is comprised of some of the women you admire most in the world, when some are your mentors and coaches, and when all of them have dared and accomplished so much in their lives, it can be daunting and intimidating to hear what they share. And if you've lived a life never quite sure that your perception of yourself is correct, it can be scary.

I will cherish each and every word shared with me that night. I will revel in the traits they saw in me and shared with me, because they acknowledged that the person I want to be is showing up visibly, beyond the dreams and goals in my mind.

One part of that journey of discovery was the unveiling of the gift of changes in the way we think.

One woman spoke of my journey of self-discovery and how, over the time we'd known each other, she'd seen me knock at the door of self-awareness over and over. Even as I'd been frustrated and thwarted in moving down my path, I kept moving into deeper awareness of who I am as a person, as a woman, as "crone." As she spoke, I realized how important the traveling of that path of self-knowledge has been for me, and how that path has paralleled my path to health and my journey as an author, a coach, and an advocate for women in menopause.

Somewhere in my mind, the second tumbler clicked into place. *5 Left.*

The Talk

The morning after my experience in that circle of women, I was given another opportunity to unwrap the mysterious gift of the changes in my brain. I was asked to participate in the inaugural *TAI Talks*, a new discussion series to highlight the differences we, as authors and thinkers, make in the world. My topic was to be, of course, menopause, and I chose to share a theme that has been common to much of my work— how we've come to be conditioned to think of menopause as a negative and how and why we should rethink that assumption.

It may not come as much of a surprise to you that I was still revising my talk a few hours before the event began. The good news was that since I was so concentrated on pulling together what I wanted to say, I didn't have much time to be nervous about the global nature of the audience!

It was only natural that, as I was extoling the blessings of menopause, the subject of this book came up. After all, I'd been spending a significant portion of my work days on it for weeks.

The last tumbler clicked into place. *11 Right.*

And I knew the answer. I saw the gift of brain fog as this sentence came into focus: *What if brain fog is a way to focus us, to hone our sight on what's important, to let go of the thousand and one trivial tasks of our days?*

The "Open"

The lock opened—like the door to Ali Baba's cave—on a treasure trove: the gifts of my changing brain. Let's take a closer look at those treasures.

The First Gift. The first gift is the gift of *examination*. Like when we're walking in the forest on a foggy day, we can only see so far when we're experiencing brain fog. And so we must slow down and examine what is close to us, look carefully at the details, and review our lives and ourselves unflinchingly. That helps us decide what to keep, what to embrace, and what to let go.

Marie Kondo wrote one of the most popular books of the past couple of years, *The Life Changing Magic of Tidying Up*, in which she wrote about decluttering our surroundings by deciding, for each and every object, whether it has a purpose and whether it brings us delight. While I'm not a complete fan of her work (I feel too attached to too many things that don't delight me but are supremely useful), there's definitely something to be said for using her method to examine the way we clutter up our lives.

When we pause and reflect on who we've been all along the journey, and consider who we'd like to be in the next phase of our lives, we get to decide whether the lessons we learned in the past still serve us, still delight us. We get to decide whether each "truth" we thought we knew longs to be kept in a place of honor in our life now or is simply a memory for the scrapbook of selfie heirlooms.

Or perhaps the lens through which we learned and continued to view life was distorted and, through examination, we've learned to see more clearly. We can do this consciously. There are pieces of our lives that we can "thank for their service" and let go. Sometimes, those feel like the simple things, beliefs like "mom is responsible for cleaning up every day." Does that belief still feel good? Is the person who has that belief still the person you want to be? Or is it time to delegate, to share the tasks of running the household with everyone who lives in the house?

Sometimes, the shifts are more profound. The belief that I always came last, always took the crushed piece of cake or the part of the pie that had lost the crust, was a big one for me. It turns out that it's sitting there at the bottom of the "unlaundered belief" pile for most of the women I work with, too. We stand to the side, holding the jackets and the souvenir bags, while our spouses and children ride the roller coasters (or the merry-go-rounds—your choice). We cancel our workouts or coffee dates with our friends so that we can provide yet one more ride for our children and their friends or attend yet more boring corporate events with our spouses.

That was an unexamined belief for me, one I inherited from my mom, my aunts, and my grandmother. It was a belief I saw modeled by my husband's mother. In order to be able to truly care for myself, to invest in myself, I had to look at that belief, to examine it and decide that I had the right to self-care. And I had the right to ask others to put my needs first on occasion.

Lest you get caught in the "who am I to be so selfish trap" when putting your own needs first, ask yourself two questions. The first question: "What am I modeling for younger women, especially my daughters?" We tell our girls they can go out and do amazing work in the world, and then we model "but only once you've fed everyone and done the dishes." The second question: "What will I have left if I never get anything back in return?" I'm sure you've heard the concept of *filling the well*. It's important to do now, in this time of your life. Truth be told, the well may fill a little slower now.

The Second Gift. The second gift is that of *perspective*. Remember that thing we were talking about? How it's become so much harder to move fluidly from chore to chore and task to task and look back at the end of the day and see a trail of accomplishment? People call it multitasking, but it's truly "serial tasking." It's much more likely—after a day of flitting from thing to thing, walking into rooms and wondering why we're there, starting and restarting and *restarting* our chores because we've forgotten what state we left things in—that we look back to see a path littered with half-done tasks, abandoned chores, and forgotten assignments.

For many of us, that's so contrary to who we were that we feel embarrassed and inept. However, our daily to-do list, when seen through the lens of menopause, might seem a bit different. Perhaps we're now better suited to concentration, to selecting the important tasks and then delegating, streamlining, or discarding the rest.

Here's another perspective shift. For most of our adult lives, estrogen informs how we think. Women were designed to work in community, to work together with other women to create lives that support and nourish each other. We're more socially aware than the hunters, the men of the tribe, more able to multitask; and our brains' communication centers are more active. But the hunters, the men, of our tribe? They had to be single-minded, and maybe even solitary, to follow the trails of the animals they hunted.

But then our estrogen levels drop, and we lose our natural edge for creating and living in community. Now we have the opportunity to think the way men have thought all their lives.

We have the chance to understand how both genders think. *We just have to get past our consternation at not thinking like we used to think.* Yes, all those things we were doing before were fabulous, and we may struggle with those ways of thinking more than we used to, but we've been given new insights into the ways the other half thinks.

The Third Gift. The third gift I rediscovered during that weekend business meeting was the gift of *focus*. When we do slow down and take our time, when we become engrossed in the moment, when we take the time to notice what we're seeing, feeling, and thinking—that's when we discover the jewels hidden in our daily existence.

Did you ever pan for gold at one of those tourist places (or for real, for that matter)? There's usually a proprietor, dressed as an old prospector, who tells stories and shows you how to work the pan in the water. You slowly wash out the dirt and debris and sift through the contents of your pan. It takes focus, concentration, and patience to control what stays in the pan and what goes. As the lighter dirt and rocks are washed out, you can begin to see glimpses of the gold, until the precious payload is all that's left in the pan.

But there's a danger point. If you glimpse that small piece of gold and don't slow down so you can be more careful about washing away the dross, the waste, you might lose that nugget of gold. In your rush, you might lose bits of treasure.

Sifting and sorting through our observations and thoughts about life is a lot like that. We have so many fleeting thoughts, so many "here-and-gone" ideas, that it's often not until we take the time to concentrate on *just one thing* that we find the gold in our pan. This is the gift of focus.

Your Gift is Waiting

These gifts of the way my brain changed—this ability to get in close and examine what was calling for my attention, this perspective on the ways people think and how our minds work, this focus on what's really important in my life—includes sharing them with you. This time of your life can be so special, so magical, so important. If you've found this book, you may still be wondering how, with all of the bizarre changes and symptoms that are happening to you, I can possibly make that claim. Don't I know what you're going through? Don't I know how scared you are?

Yes, I do. Because, not too long ago, I was right there, in the same fog you find yourself in now. These gifts I just talked about? They really aren't new in my life, but writing this chapter gave me a chance to re-examine them and find a new way to talk about them.

Now I'd like to show you how to find your own gifts.

Chapter Two

What Did I Come in Here For?

I worked with Nancy recently on a host of issues about menopause. She originally sought out my help with anxiety and depression, but as we were talking, it became clear that the thing that scared her the most was the way her thinking, her brain, was changing. Like I used to, Nancy had a job that required her to think for most of the day, and she was used to juggling a million responsibilities.

When Nancy and I started talking about that, she explained that she easily lost track of what she was doing and became distracted by whatever it was that people were asking of her, and even had trouble sometimes chasing her most interesting thought of the moment. In her high-demand job, that meant she found herself scrambling to get her tasks done on time with the quality she expected of herself, and that was something she'd never faced before.

On top of that, she was forgetting things. Nancy used to be one of those people others envy: You told her something and she never lost track of it. She was always organized, always on top of it. But lately, she told me, if she didn't write it down right away, it was gone. Maybe something would remind her in time, but maybe not. She'd forgotten promises to meet friends for drinks, driven by the grocery store without remembering to pick up the short list of items she needed, and arrived at meetings only to be reminded that she was the one who was supposed to put together the agenda—except she'd forgotten to do it.

And then there was the "forgetting names thing." And the "forgetting words thing." Nancy told me rather proudly that her dad had taught her at a young age how to remember people's names and how important it was to use their names when talking with them. All through her adult life, Nancy had been known for remembering people and their names. It was the one skill for connecting with people that she'd felt safe in. Now, however, she wished for nothing more than "name tags for everyone." She said she even wanted to tattoo her husband's name on his forehead!

The "words thing" was similar—getting halfway through a sentence and the word she wanted was gone. She would fumble and stumble and finally come up with a substitute, but much of her communication at home had become about "whatchamacallits" and "you know, the thingy," sometimes accompanied by rather comical hand gestures.

As we talked, I found myself nodding my head along with every story and description. Nancy's complaints and fears were so familiar! I'd had every last one of them myself, as a part of my own journey.

Nancy was terrified that she was losing her mind or that she had early onset Alzheimer's, and it was fueling her anxiety. I promised her that we'd change the way she thought about thinking.

The Symptoms

There are dozens of symptoms of menopause, because the changing hormone levels affect every cell of your body. Because they change every cell, they change how other hormone-producing organs work. And that changes physiological systems that you wouldn't expect to be related to your reproductive system and menopause.

Adding to the unexpectedness of the symptoms, no one tells you what to expect. Often, even the people (even your medical professionals) you do ask about it don't consider menopause to be the cause of those symptoms. If they do tell you that menopause is involved, they don't tell you how and why it's doing that to you.

In this chapter, I want to explain the symptoms I consider to be *thinking symptoms*, ways our thinking changes and sometimes malfunctions. We'll talk about how and why our thinking changes, and how to tell the difference between what you're feeling and the more dangerous changes that affect some people as they age.

There are three primary symptoms under this umbrella of thinking symptoms: *brain fog, easy distractibility*, and *memory loss*. Here's the thing about menopause—everyone's experience is personal and unique. What's happening to me may not be the same as what's going on for you. Then, too, we use different terms to explain what we're experiencing. If I'm using terms that don't grab you right away, keep reading through the descriptions and see if another one resonates with you. Or just call it "my memory thingy." Whatever works for you.

There are changes that affect our emotions—things like mood swings, anxiety, and depression—that I'm not covering in this book. But, if you're affected in the cognitive area, the broad categories of thinking symptoms should cover what you're experiencing. (If your symptoms are drastically different, would you let me know? I'm interested.)

Brain Fog

Brain fog feels to me like walking through the world without being there. When I've experienced it, I get to the end of the day and don't have a clue as to what I've done all day. There's been nothing memorable, nothing important, nothing that I cared about in the whole day. If I could figure out or remember what I've done, I'd realize that I haven't actually accomplished anything, though I may have been busy all day.

I've been "calling it in."

Brain fog is by no means a clinical diagnosis. It's simply a description of how you experience the world. Brain fog is the inability to think clearly. You feel like you are literally walking around in a fog. The world is black and white and gray; the colors are gone. Things at a distance are in soft focus.

You may not feel like doing much. You may feel an inability to concentrate that feels more like not caring. It can feel like depression, like you don't want to do anything, but if you sit with it for a few minutes, you'll likely realize that it's more like that walk in the woods I described in Chapter One—your focus wants to narrow down and zero in.

If you went to your doctor about the brain fog, the diagnosis would be something vague like "chronic cognitive and mood problems." Depending on the doctor's perspective, and which specialty she practiced, you might get a recommendation to eat healthier and exercise more, a prescription for Xanax or Prozac, or an admonition to "just get over it." But, deep in your heart or your gut, you feel that there's something real going on. It's more than just "all in your head" and you're not making a big deal out of nothing. And, being dismissed like that doesn't feel right at all.

Is It Depression?

Brain fog feels a lot like depression and, depending on who you talk to, you can allow yourself to become convinced that it is, indeed, depression, and you need to take antidepressants to deal with it. It's possible that you really are depressed. Women in menopause who've never been clinically depressed can develop depression. But is it really clinical depression?

If I were to list the symptoms of depression, you'd probably go, "Check, check, yup, got that one, too." And if I were to list the symptoms of menopause, you'd get the same list. So I'm going to give you a means to help determine if what you're experiencing is depression or menopause.

My suggestion for discerning what's going on is based on whether you can "snap out of it." I don't mean "pull yourself up by your bootstraps, bucko," but whether joy is accessible to you, hidden beneath what seems like depression.

So, here's what you do. You can do this by yourself or with a friend who's not part of your daily routine but whose company you enjoy. Choose an activity you've always loved but haven't done recently. It could be going to a museum or to a movie, window-shopping at an upscale location, or taking a whitewater rafting trip. This shouldn't be a bucket list item; it should be something you already know you like. Arrange your schedule so you're not leaving pressing matters undone, and then go do it. Let yourself go while you're doing it. When you've done it, ask yourself, *Did I enjoy it? Did I have fun? Was I present in the moment?*

If you didn't start to feel connected to yourself in that situation, you may want to consider whether talking with a professional about depression might be a good idea. But, if you had a positive, feel-good experience, you may be experiencing brain fog from menopause.

Either way, whether it's depression or menopause brain fog or both, the information in the next few chapters will help you recover your mental sharpness and personal shine.

Easy Distractibility

My all-time favorite depiction of this thinking symptom comes from the wonderful movie *Up*, in which the talking dog, Dug, is distracted over and over from the task at hand. A movement in his peripheral vision creates instant distraction and he turns and exclaims, "Squirrel!"

If you've experienced that feeling, you know exactly what I mean. You start a task like, say, cleaning up the living room. You take a couple of leftover glasses into the kitchen. While you're putting them in the dishwasher, you notice a plant that needs watering, so you give it a drink. That makes you remember the plant in your bedroom, so you take it some water. While you're in the bedroom, you see the book you fell asleep reading last night and wonder what happened to the heroine, so you stop to read a chapter. The phone rings, so you answer it and need to dash to your desk to check your computer about a payment. Facebook messenger beeps, so you check a message from a friend, and now you're down the FB rabbit-hole. At the end of the day, the vacuum cleaner is still sitting in the middle of the living room, unused, the dishwasher door is open, the bedroom plant is dying from lack of water, the bills aren't paid, and you're playing solitaire on the computer.

It can happen in the workplace, too. You begin working on a task and someone asks you a question. Or you get called away to a meeting. Or the phone rings. When you finally get back to what you were doing, you've lost your place and you need to start over. When interruptions happen over and over during the day, you get to the end of your day and feel like you've gotten nothing done.

A year ago, you'd have never been distracted, or you'd have circled back to every task and completed it, and accomplished so much more in your day. You wonder where your focus and ability to concentrate have gone. You were the queen of multitasking, but now you wonder if this isn't some bizarre form of attention deficit disorder (ADD) that occurs to women in midlife.

Is It ADD?

In a word, no. Unless you've been highly distractible all your life, this is probably not what's happening. Besides, there's no evidence that ADD or ADHD (attention deficit hyperactive disorder) are disorders that first appear in adulthood.

What's happening is that the parts of your brain that deal with multitasking are no longer being stimulated by estrogen, and so you really aren't able to multitask in the same way you used to. But you're in the habit of multitasking, so you continue to live with that pattern. Your brain *has* changed, and the way you do things is no longer efficient for the new way you think. (In the next chapter, I'll share some of the science behind this, and then we'll get into the real issues—what you can do about it.)

Memory Loss

Memory loss as a thinking symptom seems pretty common, too. You walk into a room and forget why you're there. Or you can't find your glasses, and then find them a few days later in the freezer. Or you're writing an email and can't find the right word. Or (my personal non-favorite) you can't remember someone's name, even though you've known her forever.

While those all may feel like senior moments, they can also be pretty scary. The first time it happens, you might wonder if you've had a mini-stroke (also called a *transient ischemic attack* or *TIA*). As incidents like that keep occurring, you begin to wonder if it's Alzheimer's. Fear sets in and you start analyzing every action and thought, and it seems to get worse.

Is It a Stroke? Is It Alzheimer's?

While the symptoms can be terrifying and there are so many similarities between the memory lapses we experience in menopause and Alzheimer's or a stroke, for most of us, the symptoms are a result of the changes of menopause and normal aging. Occasionally, they signal that we need to pay attention to our brain health in the ways that I'll be talking about in the rest of the book. But, just to put you at ease, let's talk about some of the symptoms of these more serious problems.

Symptoms of a TIA. A *TIA*, or *transient ischemic attack*, is a temporary blockage of a blood vessel in the brain. The symptoms are similar to a stroke, but last for a short amount of time (less than five minutes, usually, less than one). The symptoms include numbness in one side of the body or face, confusion, vision trouble in one or both eyes, severe headache, and loss of coordination or balance.

A TIA usually resolves in less than 24 hours. A series of TIAs could result in gradual decline in mental and neurological function and could be a prelude to a stroke, so if it happens, you do need to get medical help immediately. The difference between a series of TIAs and the kind of memory loss we're talking about is that there's usually an incident that you can identify as this type of mini-stroke. The little memory blips of menopause (or even of normal "happens to everyone" distractions)—a forgotten word or a name or a misplaced item—don't have other symptoms with them.

Symptoms of a stroke. An actual stroke is a much more severe blockage of blood circulation. It is distinguished from a TIA by its severity and duration. It is a life-threatening emergency and needs medical attention immediately.

The protocol for determining a stroke and the need for treatment is in the acronym FAST: *F*acial drooping, which usually affects one side of the face, *A*rm weakness, on the same side as the drooping, *S*peech difficulties—inability to speak clearly, often with confusion, and *T*ime, which means that prompt action is critical.

It is important to reach emergency treatment as soon as possible in the case of either a TIA or a stroke.

Symptoms of Alzheimer's. The symptoms listed in the 2014 fact sheet of the Alzheimer's Association (www.alz.org/downloads/Facts_Figures_2014.pdf) include memory loss (including names and events), confusion, challenges in problem solving, misplacing things, difficulty in understanding spatial relationships, decreased judgment, social withdrawal, and changes in mood and personality. The Alzheimer's Association emphasizes that all of these symptoms may begin gradually and progress.

Okay, stop! Don't have a panic attack yet!

Is it Alzheimer's or is it menopause?

So far, you're diagnosing yourself with early onset Alzheimer's and are ready to check yourself in to long-term care, right? Just stop it! Stop freaking out and thinking the worst. Yes, it happens. Yes, it's scary. Yes, it could be happening to you.

But. But the incidence of early onset Alzheimer's, defined as happening earlier than at age 65, is less than four percent of the total cases of Alzheimer's. And the total incidence of dementia is about one in nine for those over 65 (and it's progressive—a far greater percentage of those over the age of 80 have dementia than those between 65 and 80). That works out to be about a 0.3% (three in one thousand, including both men and women) incidence of early onset Alzheimer's. On the other hand, the percentage of women who are experiencing at least perimenopausal changes comes close to 100 percent by age 55. Therefore, the likelihood that the changes you are experiencing are from menopause is much higher than the chance of early onset Alzheimer's.

Then there's the belief you may have that decline is inevitable from Alzheimer's. As research continues on dementia, however, it's becoming clear that many cases of Alzheimer's are treatable and that changes in cognition can be limited. There is still no definitive test for Alzheimer's or other forms of dementia without an autopsy (really, that's not an option at this point—I'm not volunteering for one), so there's no way to tell whether what you are experiencing is Alzheimer's or menopause. Wouldn't you rather assume that you are going to be able to influence what's going on in your brain?

I'm not telling you not to discuss this with your doctor. I'm only telling you that over the next few chapters we're going to talk about the changes in your brain from menopause and how you can maximize brain health at this time in your life. Those practices are the same as the ones most functional medicine practitioners would advise to promote the least decline as you age, overall.

Wouldn't you do something about the brain fog, whatever it's from, rather than just worry about it?

Other Causes of Brain Fog

Before we get to the changes you can make, I want to talk about some of the other conditions for which brain fog is a symptom. Some of these are pretty common and may be related to menopause. Others are diseases or disorders for which brain fog is a symptom. In general, I advise my clients to do specific research on their own symptoms if they are concerned that what they are experiencing is beyond the symptoms of menopause.

Related (Or Potentially Related) Causes

Lack of sleep. Insomnia can be a huge cause of brain fog, lack of concentration, and memory lapses. And, yes, menopausal hormone shifts can be a big reason you aren't sleeping. I cover a number of fixes for insomnia in Chapter Seven.

Stress. Stress can also create brain fog. The more acute the stress, the more likely it is that the more primitive, reactive parts of your brain are in control, while the rational parts aren't. Chapter Eight covers ways of managing stress and thereby making it easier to think more clearly.

Nutritional issues. Certain vitamin and mineral deficiencies make it harder to think, as do dehydration and lack of protein. Food sensitivities can make thinking more difficult, as can type 2 diabetes and its precursors. Menopausal changes seem to exacerbate gluten sensitivities as well as increase the possibility of insulin resistance.

Thyroid issues. Brain fog can be a symptom of low thyroid hormone levels, which are often triggered by the changes of menopause or by the high cortisol levels that accompany menopause.

Yeast infections (candida). Yeast infections can be quite common in menopause, and often recur, because they aren't completely flushed from the system. Look at not only the symptoms of vaginal yeast infections, but also symptoms of thrush or systemic yeast infections.

Non-Related Causes

Medications. If you're on any medications, read the inserts that come with the medication or look it up on WebMD or another reputable site. Many medications have brain fog-type side effects. If this is the case for you, you can speak with your prescribing physician about changing medications or changing dosages.

Environmental toxins. Some women have sensitivities to household cleaners and chemicals or molds that are in their daily environment, and all of us have a threshold beyond which these start to affect us.

Lyme disease or other brain parasites. Increasingly, brain fog is being seen as a long-term consequence of parasitic diseases that eventually attack the brain. These diseases are typically extremely difficult to diagnose, especially if you don't live in an area that is known for the presence of the disease.

Fibromyalgia. Fibromyalgia is a condition characterized by all-over pain and aching. Symptoms also include crushing fatigue, unrefreshing sleep, cognitive issues, abdominal and digestive symptoms, and sensory sensitivity. Fibromyalgia can be aggravated by menopause, so it's hard to tell the difference sometimes.

Lupus. Lupus is a serious autoimmune disorder. Chronic and severe inflammation is its primary characteristic. It is often distinguished by a rash that has a "butterfly shape" across the face, and it often involves multiple organs and body systems.

Chronic Fatigue Syndrome (CFS). Chronic fatigue syndrome is a term used to describe a condition where there's no other diagnosis, but there's a pattern of crashing fatigue and soreness and non-specific "unwellness," without any diagnosable condition. Although many doctors want to think of this as a psychological condition, it seems to be one of many physical conditions that aren't well understood. Adrenal fatigue may be a symptom of CFS.

Multiple Sclerosis (MS). While brain fog is a symptom of MS, MS often strikes before perimenopause typically begins (typical onset for MS is between ages 20 and 40). Other symptoms include numbness and muscle weakness, clumsiness, and lack of coordination and balance. These aren't generally symptoms of menopause and may be indicative of something more serious.

Before You Panic

Yes, brain fog can be a symptom of a number of disorders, some of them serious. But remember that menopause is a natural change that happens to 100 percent of the women that age into it. Sooner or later, it happens to all of us women, if we live long enough (for most of us, it happens between 45 and 60). Those other conditions, especially the serious ones, happen with far less frequency. Most of them are diagnosed in less than two-tenths of one percent (less than two in 1,000) of the entire population, men and women included.

Talking to Your Doctor

Brain changes can be frightening. I totally get that. Unlike many other symptoms of menopause, there are a number of real and debilitating conditions that can show up as brain fog or confusion or distractibility. So, if you are at all concerned about what's going on with you, I encourage you to speak with your doctor and create a plan to monitor and/or diagnose what's happening with you.

But you also don't have to be scared while you are dealing with the medical system either. Here are the steps that I recommend.

1. Relax and fire Dr. Google. Stop thinking about every negative symptom this might be. It probably is menopause brain. Worrying will only make it worse.

2. Collect your "evidence." Write down examples of the kinds of changes you are experiencing and how often they are occurring. Ask others who are close to you whether they've noticed changes and what kinds of changes they've seen.

3. Make your appointment. If my clients ask me about it, I suggest that they see a doctor or practitioner who knows them—either their primary care doctor or their gynecologist. The more the doctor understands about menopause and about you, the better. Going to a neurologist without talking to a generalist first is like talking to a carpenter who only has a hammer about a plumbing problem—to that carpenter, everything's a nail.

4. Take someone with you. A second set of ears in the doctor's office is always a good idea. This is especially true if it's possible that the diagnosis may be upsetting. It also helps to write down

your questions beforehand, so that you'll be more likely to get the answers you need.

5.   Explain yourself carefully. I always suggest that the first words you use to describe your issue are "I think I'm in menopause" and tell them why you think that. If the doctor dismisses that as irrelevant, you might want to consider getting a second opinion.

6.   Make sure you get the answers you need. Doctors can be busy people and they can think they are busier than they are. Get the answers you need and have a plan to follow-up with the doctor, if needed.

The Next Steps

I hope this chapter has helped you figure out in that the symptoms you've been experiencing are pretty common and that they're very likely not indicators of major disease or the imminent demise of your ability to function. And that's a really good thing.

But, knowing that these are common symptoms doesn't help that much, does it? Even knowing that there can be upsides to these brain things may not be very comforting. Comfort is on its way, though, so keep reading.

What I want to do next is give you an explanation of what's going on and why the changes in your reproductive system create changes in the way you think. It can be good to understand what's going on, but if science isn't really your thing, and you want to get right to fixing things, feel free to skip over the next chapter (you can always come back to it if you want).

In the six chapters after the science chapter, I'll share some of the best techniques I know and use with my clients to help them get back to thinking like themselves. Or even better.

Chapter Three
My Inner Science Geek Speaks

—•—

O h, so you want a story? Well, okay. But this one isn't strictly factual—it's the way I imagine your many-times remote ancestresses must have lived...

Una and Madja were members of a hunter-gather tribe, living a precarious existence in a post-Ice Age era. Una was still a young woman, while Madja was older, past her child-bearing years. She no longer bled on her monthly cycle. Madja was a rarity. Most women died in child-birth or from famine, but Madja had given birth to several children and raised two of them to adulthood. She was considered a "wise woman" and knew much about herbs and healing. No one could remember ever being part of the tribe when Madja wasn't there.

Una had many responsibilities in her daily life. She and the other women her age would travel the area around their current camping site to look for berries, fruits, herbs, and even root vegetables. They cleaned and cured the meats that the men, who were the hunters, brought home, and even participated in the massive hunts that provided a good deal of their winter provisions. Una had a small child and spent time each day nursing him. All of the women were constantly on the watch for the toddlers and the youngsters, who were always getting into everything.

The women were also responsible for the protecting the camp from the wild animals that tried to prey on the children or on the precious stores. They also guarded against other tribes, who might come raiding for furs and stores or try to carry off young women as trophies (and, for, well, you know). Since the women had to defend the children, they couldn't simply flee, and because they were often less strong than their attackers, they had to work together to provide the defenses they needed.

Una had a mate, Beorg, who was a superior provider, and when he was not gone with the hunters, she did her best to keep him happy and content, so that he wouldn't abandon her for some other woman of the tribe. Una's life was filled with keeping her man happy, working and socializing with her "sisters," and doing the many diverse tasks required to keep the camp safe and productive.

Madja's life was a little different. Since she was past her fertile years, no man was really interested in her, and ever since her mate, Mindal, had been killed in a hunting accident, she had been alone in camp. But her skills with herbs, gained as an apprentice to an earlier wise woman, meant that she was still a valuable member of the tribe. She spent much of her time alone or in the company of an apprentice (she had her eye on Una, but Una was still a young and attractive woman mostly interested in her family). Madja gathered herbs, made poultices and tinctures, and treated the wounds and illnesses of the tribe. She served as a midwife for women going through childbirth. She was a valued, even revered, member of the tribe.

But, for all her commitment and competence, Madja was cautious. She still remembered the fate of Naona, the woman who had taught Madja's mentor. Naona had rejected the advances of one of the tribal elders. A short time later, the tribe had camped in a new location and several members had fallen sick. When two of them died, Naona was blamed for not saving them and shunned by the tribe.

Madja was grateful that the elders seemed to support her, but she knew that they could be fickle, and she did not have the protection of a hunter and the responsibility for young children. She continued to build her relationships with the younger women of the tribe, even though she found that to be tiring. She simply wasn't as interested in their company as she had once been. She persisted in sharing her knowledge, though, because she wanted them to know as much as possible and because she hoped that they would protect her if she ever needed it.

The Difference Between Men and Women

What does the story of Una and Madja have to do with anything? Why do I bother thinking about the way the way they lived way back when? What does it have to do with how we live today?

It all comes down to the differences between men and women.

If you think back to biology class, or to trying to tutor your high-schooler through his or her biology class, you might be thinking that the difference between men and women all boils down to DNA, to genetics. Men have an X and a Y chromosome, and women have two X chromosomes, right? That's what determines it all.

Well, yes and no. The yes part is that when an egg is fertilized, it has half of the 26 chromosome pairs. The 26th pair half of the egg is always an "X" chromosome. The sperm that fertilizes the egg brings the other half of the 26 pairs. The 26th chromosome is either an "X" or a "Y." If it's an X, the baby will have all the physical accoutrements of a female (uterus, ovaries, etc.). If it's a Y, it's a boy and gets those other things (penis, testicles, prostate, etc.). So far, so good.

The fetus's brain is, in the very beginning, not distinguished by sex. For the first two trimesters, the baby's brain is the same whether it's a boy or a girl. Then, in the last trimester, the brain gets a massive infusion of either testosterone or of estrogen. That's when the differentiation begins.

Louanne Brezidene, in her book *The Female Brain*, explains that this initial burst of estrogen means that baby girls are much more oriented to their mothers' faces. They are more communicative and provide more feedback to their mothers and, in effect, reward their mothers for interacting with them.

That's only the beginning. Girls appear to get an additional shot of estrogen to their brains before they are two, accounting for many of the differences observed in how boys and girls play. For example, girls tend to cooperate more, laying out the parameters of their games with their playmates in elaborate sets of rules. Think about two girls playing house—"You be the mommy, I'll be the daddy, and Spot, the dog, will be our little boy." The rules alone can take most of the playtime.

Then comes a period when everything calms down hormonally. Girls go about the business of learning and doing, as do boys. Boosted by the earlier shots of estrogen, girls thrive in the classroom, where communication skills are highly rewarded. Boys, with their higher levels of testosterone driving them to higher levels of aggression and impulsivity, are much more likely to be diagnosed as hyperactive and are less interested in sitting still and learning.

That's how it goes until puberty, when everything changes for both genders. High levels of estrogen in girls, now young women, flood the centers for communication and socialization, focusing them firmly on babies, boys, and biology (their own). Boys, flooded with testosterone, find competition to be their central focus; although action is still an important driver for them, they also begin to be more able to concentrate and focus on the task at hand.

Physical Differences in Male and Female Brains

Interestingly enough, the brain structures are actually different between men and women, supporting the ways that women and men think differently. For example, women have verbal centers in both hemispheres of their brains, while men generally have only one verbal center. This means that women tend to use more words more frequently than men do. It also results in there being more connectivity and communication between the hemispheres of the brain. Since the left and right hemispheres do have different functions, this may explain why women are often much more capable of articulating not only thoughts, but feelings as well.

When it comes to memory, women have a more connections to a more highly developed hippocampus, which is responsible for human sensory and emotive memories. This means that women notice more details during an event and remember them more vividly. Women, in general, have a higher number of connections in their brains (more "white matter") and higher blood flow. In particular, the area responsible for specific types of concentration, the *cingulate gyrus*, is much more active for women, meaning that women tend to "chew on" emotional experiences much more than men do.

Another area of the brain, the *frontopolar prefrontal cortex*, which is responsible for multitasking, appears to be more developed in women than in men. This corresponds well to the observations that women are better able to switch from one task to another—the famous multitasking ability of women.

Oxytocin is a neurotransmitter (a brain hormone) that makes us feel super good, and women are more reactive to oxytocin than men.

Oxytocin is released in significant quantities when snuggling with a mate, a cat, or sometimes just with a cup of tea. But it really goes into hyper-drive when we connect with a baby. In fact, breast feeding releases massive quantities of this hormone.

Women also react differently to danger than men do. The amygdala, the part of the brain that's responsible for immediate reactions to danger, is more developed in men, so men appear to be more reactive to danger. Estrogen appears to modulate or dampen the effects of the stress hormone cortisol. This means that women don't react to stress as much as men do. There's also some evidence that women react differently under stress, too. Their response is not "fight-or-flight," but "tend-and-befriend." Women in high stress situations have a greater tendency to care for the helpless and to work together to solve the problem.

Those are only some of the observed differences in men and women's brains. I want to emphasize that for any difference in the way the sexes think, there's a continuum. So, even if that old thing about men being better at science and math is true in the absolute (I'm not saying it is), that doesn't mean that some women aren't better than all but a handful (or less) of men. The same is true in reverse. There are men who are better communicators than all but a few women. But it's important to look at the generalities so that we can understand, first, why they exist and, second, what happens to us in menopause.

Why the Differences Exist

Some of what follows is speculation. Since they weren't actually studying this stuff when Madja and Una were around and they didn't leave many records, we don't know for sure how they actually lived. But let's look at some of the reasons that women, especially women in their childbearing years, think the way they do.

In a hunter-gatherer culture, women have a greater need for men and for other women than men have need for women. Compared to other species, humans have a fairly long gestation period and are more incapable of hunting during the last part of pregnancy. Also, human infants are incapable of taking care of themselves for much longer than most mammals. In most cases, a woman would starve or be killed long before she was able to raise a child to the point it could be left alone while she hunted. Men, on the other hand, could remain largely self-sufficient once they were old enough to hunt.

Since women needed the community around them more than men did, it seems only natural that they developed the ability to create it. Their verbal abilities and socializing skills were needed to draw others to them and to create the connections that held the tribe together and that kept them safe. While the (male) hunters needed the aggression and even the competitiveness to chase down and slaughter prey, the women needed to work together to protect the camp and the children, to preserve the food, and to create the means of sheltering and clothing the tribe.

Multitasking, too, was a prized ability for those early women. Cooking and caring for children weren't "full-time" tasks, but they were (and are) tasks that demand full attention at critical points. For example, when a child toddles near an open fire, you must stop and attend to the child without delay. The same goes for a stew that's about to boil over. Neither interruption needs to take long, but it means that the woman must be able to move seamlessly from one task to another and still complete them.

Then there's the stress response. You can see how helpful it is for women to react more calmly, to protect children and sick people, and to work with others in times of danger. Because children are so important to the women of the tribe, they work to protect them. Because women are physically smaller and weaker than the men of marauding tribes and perhaps than predatory animals, they had to work together to find the solutions to those threats.

Brain Changes at Menopause

Hypothesizing that the primary difference between the way men and women's brains work is the amount of estrogen present in the brain is helpful in understanding the way menopause changes us. Again, there's little hard evidence of these statements, because research in this area is just getting started, but I hope you'll find that these hypotheses help you understand more about what's happening as your estrogen levels drop.

First, let's look at that verbal fluency thing. Without the stimulation of estrogen, our verbal centers don't operate at peak efficiency anymore. Secondary verbal centers may become less available to us, and so we find ourselves hunting for words. Because we're not as stimulated in the social centers, and because we don't make as rapid connections between the verbal centers and the centers responsible for things like remembering names, those faculties don't work as well as they used to.

Memories may not be created as easily and, even when they are, they may not be recorded in our brains as sharply as they once were. Details may be lacking, as well as emotional content.

Multitasking becomes more difficult.

A change that most women find confusing is that we become more introverted and less "people-pleasing" as we go through menopause. That makes sense now, doesn't it? When estrogen pushes us at puberty to connect with others, especially males, in menopause, the levels of estrogen fall, and its absence encourages us to develop a new relationship, not with others, but with ourselves.

Finally, there's that change in handling cortisol. While the focus of this book is not on the emotional changes that may accompany menopause, I want to bring this particular change up because it can be so scary and make us feel so irrational.

The cortisol reaction in your body can feel like anxiety or panic— racing heartbeat, shallow, rapid breathing, tense muscles, increased sensory input, and even internal trembling can make us feel like the world is about to end. If you've never experienced anxiety before, you may not even know what's happening at first. If you have, you know exactly what's happening. Either way, you're looking for something or someone to blame, for something to be scared of. You can put yourself into an escalating cycle of anxiety attacks, because you experience the stimulus of the cortisol and so you become afraid, which makes you more afraid, and so on and so on.

When I work with women around anxiety, our first priority is to understand that this change is physical rather than emotional, and that—even if their bodies create a feeling of anxiety—if they can manage their thinking, anxiety doesn't need to become a problem.

Is There Any Hope at All?

A few weeks ago, I was working with a woman around these issues. Let's call her Belinda. Belinda was a bit of a science geek, too, and she kept asking more questions about the ways her brain was changing, and so I kept going a little deeper. After about 40 minutes of that (which is more than many of my clients can stand of physiology), she said, "Boy, that's pretty bleak. Isn't there anything *good* happening in my brain?"

It occurs to me that you might be thinking that very thing right now. I was writing this chapter yesterday and when I got to this point, I had to take a break because I was so deep in the negative feelings that can arise around the changes that I couldn't even remember what I'd been planning to write about the positives! Fortunately, I woke up this morning remembering what I needed to tell you.

The Way the New You Thinks

Yes, losing your ability to multitask seems terrible. As do all those memory lapses, including forgetting people's names right after you meet them. And what's with that whole "now I'm an introvert" thing? Some of us even retreat from our families, our friends, and our community.

Then here I come, telling you all this dire stuff and telling you to consider it a gift.

I still say that. Yes, we think differently now. But different isn't necessarily worse. Let me show you why.

For the last 25 to 30 years, you've concentrated on making things run smoothly—your home, your job, your family. Maybe you've raised children. If you had babies in your life, you probably had baby-brain fog far worse than what you're experiencing now, but you were getting such amazing shots of oxytocin from all that cuddle time that you don't even remember how bad it was.

Maybe you've had a career, or maybe a job, or maybe you were one of those amazing stay-at-home moms on whom the rest of us depend to keep the world running right (I'm not kidding here; if it weren't for the stay-at-home mom, we'd all be in a world of hurt). Multitasking was absolutely critical to getting through your day.

Most of us have enjoyed being, to whatever extent we were, social people—meeting and interacting with people on the job, through our children's activities, and in our community. It not only puzzles us that we don't feel as connected now, but it saddens us as well.

So, what are the upsides of this?

First of all, there's the ability to concentrate. You may stop to stare at those words, because you feel like you've absolutely lost the ability to get anything done (as I said, one of the symptoms is that you feel like you've acquired a case of ADD), but what really happened is that you've lost the ability to multitask, and you're so used to doing that well that when you, by habit, try to keep operating by multitasking, it feels like you're wandering around the house getting nothing done. (By the way, that crossing-the-threshold-into-a-different-room-and-not-knowing-why-you're-there thing is called *the doorway effect*, and men have been doing it all their lives. They just assume they didn't come in to the new room to do anything in particular.)

Yes, adapting to this new way your brain works requires training yourself to focus on a single task. And, yes, there will probably be times when you'll still feel totally scattered if you try to work like you used to. Expect a couple of burnt meals, some chores left half done, projects abandoned because you can't find any chunks of time to devote to them. But, when you concentrate on a task without breaks, you actually find yourself more productive and capable of creating amazing work.

Then there's that fogginess. What I've learned about that is exactly what I remembered on that hike in New Hampshire. When you're in a fog, you're encouraged to look at details, to examine what you can see right here. Once again, you're being urged to look at and connect with what is right in front of you, to what's closest to you. Hint: in most cases, what's closest to you is yourself.

Although it isn't strictly a thinking skill, you can explore the gift of being an introvert by choice. It's not that you don't care about other people; it's that you are now capable of caring about yourself to the same extent that you care about others. All your adult life, you have lived for other people's agendas. Even when you thought you were being selfish or self-centered, it was likely primarily because your brain was telling you that you ought to be caring more about others, and you were going against that.

Now you have a chance to examine and reexamine your own hopes, dreams, and desires. The nudges of your biology are releasing you from being a people-pleaser. You have the luxury of *choosing* what you want to do, of being who you want to be. This doesn't mean that you ignore what others want or need, but you have the choice as to the importance you'll give them in your life.

You may still have others who are dependent on you—younger children, aging parents, even grandchildren. Even so, you can choose to be the center of the world for them. That's always a choice, and it can be very fulfilling. Just know it's a choice. Kids raised in an environment where Mom is more fulfilled tend to be happier and more independent anyway.

Lastly, that verbal fluency thing? Quite honestly, I'm still working out what it means for me. As a writer, I'm never far from my thesaurus. My language is more precise because I search for the right word not only in my memory but in other sources. What do you think the advantages of decreased verbal fluency are for you?

The Return of Brain Estrogen

Another thing I discovered when I was fact-checking for this section is something that is pretty much cutting edge science. It's so new that when I contacted the researcher doing the work—Brian Kenealy of University of Wisconsin, Madison—he told me that he couldn't even answer some of my basic questions because the research hasn't been done.

The primary work his team is doing has shown that estrogen production occurs not only in the ovaries and the adrenals, but the brain also produces its own estrogen, especially in the area associated with memory (the hippocampus). They've primarily been studying what happens prior to puberty and at puberty in girls. It appears that before puberty, when the levels of circulating estrogen are low, the brain produces estrogen at a level that keeps the female brain comfortable and protected.

Then, at puberty, levels of blood estrogen (circulating from the ovaries, primarily) rise and the production of brain estrogen decreases, because it's not needed.

It's reasonable to hypothesize that as blood estrogen decreases as menopausal changes happen, brain estrogen can return. If this is true, it explains why many women only feel the effects of these brain symptoms for a short while, perhaps while brain production of estrogen gets up to speed, and then feel much sharper as post-menopause continues.

So, What Do You Do with All This?

In light of all this information, what do you do? Do you resign yourself to a few years of misery? Force everyone around you to wear nametags full-time? Get a box of kittens and become a crazy cat lady?

Absolutely not! I wrote this book to provide information, coping strategies, and ways to support your brain, so that it's in the best possible working shape it can be. In Chapter Two, we talked about "other things" that can cause or contribute to thinking symptoms. Well, by taking care of our bodies, we take care of our brains. We can reduce the effects of menopause and many of those other conditions.

Chapter Four

Hacks to Help You
Get Through Your Day

W hen I reconnected with one of my old friends on a trip through San Francisco a few years back, we dumped her pre-teen kids on her husband for the day and headed out to a "girl's day out" on Fisherman's Wharf. Amy was one of the few people I still maintained contact with from my elementary school days and, though we saw each other infrequently, we always picked up right where we left off.

This time, I was excited to tell her about the changes that had been happening in my life, the new directions my research and reading were taking me, and how I had been using it to help women going through menopause. But before I could start in on my news, she began to tell me about an old friend of ours that she had run into not long before.

We began to reminisce about our sixth-grade class, which really had been special. But, for every memory, the names were, well, gone. "Who was that boy with the red-hair? Oh, you know, he was best friends with what's-

his-name," she'd say. Or I'd say, "Remember the day that... oh, who was that? Remember? She lived over by the church where we met for Girl Scouts..."

Finally, after a few minutes of that, she said to me, "I think we're getting old. We're beginning to sound just like our mothers."

I love being handed a natural lead-in. Don't you?

I began to tell Amy all the stuff I had been finding out. She was "ahead" of me on the menopause journey at that point—already done with menopause and in her first year of post-menopause, and maybe a little grumpy about it.

"Enough with the science stuff, already," Amy cut me short. "Tell me what to do about it."

"The day-to-day stuff?" I asked.

"Yes!" she replied. "Get me through my days without forgetting to pick up the kids, or make a fool of myself at the office, or serve chicken without rice, because I forgot to buy it."

This is what I shared with her...

Make a List and Check It Twice

Nope, this isn't Santa stuff. But if you don't rely on a Day-Timer or a good calendar and note-taking app, or if you're used to switching from one to the other seamlessly, it's time to get yourself organized in a whole new way, girlfriend.

I admit that I'm not an organizer by nature. I know women who teach this stuff really well, and I take their courses and still don't get it right. So this is definitely a "do as I say, not as I do" section. The cold, hard, practical truth is that if you aren't organized, you're creating stress for yourself. That means you need to get organized in a bunch of areas.

Organize your lists. Make sure you have systems for noting the things you need to remember, whether those are appointments and daily tasks that you need to accomplish, or groceries you need to buy or things you need to do in order to prepare for a special event.

Even more importantly, *coordinate those systems.* This is where I've always gotten in trouble. I have my work list—my client appointments, my writing, my appointments with the people who work on various tasks with me—and then I have my personal list—my exercise and trips and adventures, my time with my husband and friends, my Mardi Gras krewe obligations. There are a few things that cross both lines, like my involvement in civic organizations. I still, once or twice a month, double book myself, because those areas of my life reside in separate places in my brain—and sometimes in my organizational systems.

So I am constantly looking for and creating new lists and organizational tools that *work for me.* That's a really big part of the solution. What works for me may not work for you. What works for me today might, unfortunately, not work for me tomorrow. And something better might come along. Find what works for you and stick with it until it doesn't. Then identify what's not working about it and look for something that does.

Organize your time. I like each day to be a fresh experience. I like having vast, unplanned areas on my calendar that allow me to look at what's going on in my life and my work that day and say, "I think I'd like to do *x* today." I used to be able to do that, because time didn't seem to get misplaced like a set of errant car keys.

And now it does. I can start my week by blocking out time for coaching, writing, exercising, and socializing, but if I don't allot them to specific time slots, I lose track of them.

While you're at it, cut back on the multitasking. I know that when a mental squirrel runs across your desk, you'd like to chase it, but—trust me on this—when you parse a big task into lots of little chunks, make sure they can be completed in the time you have for them and beware of distractions. Otherwise, you'll find yourself starting again, over and over and over. Make larger chunks of time available, and don't expect to be able to come back to something halfway through and pick up where you left off.

Another infinitely useful tool is alarms. Hey, smartphones were made for menopausal women, and the best thing on them, to me, are the alarms and timers. I use the timers and I pre-set daily alarms and calendar reminders and anything else I can to trigger action reminders, like to keep from forgetting that I turned on the yard sprinklers or to remember to move the laundry from the washer to the dryer or to go to an important appointment.

Alarms are not the same as notifications. Choose your alarms carefully, and turn notifications off if you can, like the dings notifying you of a new Facebook message. Emails and Facebook Messenger interruptions are great big rabbit-holes. You can get lost in them for hours. Take the time to set your notifications in such a way that you know what that buzzing is about without even needing to look at it. Oh, but do take your husband's phone calls. It's just easier that way.

Organize your space. By this I mean declutter. Yep. I said it. Me, one-half of the ultimate pack-rat couple. I say to declutter. Give your eyes and your mind less to see, to notice, to need to deal with. I truly believe that, as we age, we have way too much top-of-mind stuff—deep thinking stuff—that we need to deal with. If you look around your space and it's cluttered, it's too easy to be drawn off track.

As I look around my office this morning, for example, I see that a number of things that need to be returned to their "homes" are hanging around, because I haven't had a chance to straighten up for a couple of days. So, books I've used, shoes I've worn, and the "leftover fur" from two cats and a dog are trying to claim my attention and draw me away from writing this book.

It can be a great help to do that "a place for everything and everything in its place" thing. If you aren't there yet, it's time. It really does make things easier. Especially do this for the most important things you need when you're headed out the door—wallet, car keys, phone, glasses.

Make a Habit of Creating Habits

While we're talking about organization, let's talk about what I consider the single most useful tool to overcoming both the brain fog thing and the overwhelm we can feel from living in this crazy-busy world: creating habits. Doing things without having to decide on them every time or think too much about them takes away your need for using your brain power or your will power.

It's said that we do as much as 90% of our day, including the words we use, by habit. Sometimes, those habits are powerful positive forces in our lives. Getting out of bed at much the same hour every day, brushing our teeth, our morning routines, going to work, caring for our children and pets, kissing our spouses as they leave and when they return. These are really good things, and you probably don't have to think much about doing them.

Sometimes, though, our habits can be really negative. Habits like smoking, spending time scrolling through Facebook, playing computer solitaire, or even reading too much may be negative habits for you. Some of those are bad for our health and some are just plain bad for our lives. They get in the way of us accomplishing what we really do want to get done in our lives.

Sometimes we don't even know things are habits at all. Things like setting your purse down wherever you happen to stop first when you come in the door, so that later, when you want to leave the house, you can't find it. Or not returning to the same activity after you stop to go to the bathroom. Instead, you grab something to drink or answer the phone and then you're off in a million other directions. Or not writing down something that occurs to you while you're doing something else, so you don't remember it when you're done. Those are habits. Habits of *not* doing something. And they can be just as damaging as the bad habits of *doing* something.

There's a simple method for building habits that I'd like to share with you in brief. It was developed by B. J. Fogg of Stanford University, and I share versions of this with my clients all the time. It's a five-step process:

- **Step One:** Decide on the habit you'd like to develop and when you'd like to perform it. Limit yourself originally to one new habit a day; you can spread out from there once you've established the first habit.
- **Step Two:** Break your action down into tiny sequential steps. The first couple of steps should be so easy and quick to perform that you won't *not* do it.
- **Step Three:** Find a trigger habit. Find something you already do habitually at that time of the day so that you can chain your new habit onto it. If you can, put a reminder somewhere where you'll see it when you're doing the already established habit.
- **Step Four:** Do it! Chain the first tiny step of your new habit to the old habit.
- **Step Five:** (This is the most important step!) Recognize what you've done and celebrate it. Pat yourself on the back, jump up and down, do a silly little dance. Go overboard with your self-praise. *This* is what establishes the link in your head that you've accomplished something, and that helps the habit to form.

Once the first part of the new habit is established, build on that until you have the whole habit built. Depending on what the habit is, it could take a couple weeks or even months to establish the new habit. Easy habits may take only weeks—setting up the coffee machine the night before, for example—while more complex habits that are potentially annoying to get used to, like working out every morning, will take longer and have more steps.

Sit Back and Relax

Wouldn't it feel nice to know that you didn't have anything to do right now. That you could take a nap, or sit back and daydream, or take a walk? Think about how you'd feel if you had that kind of space in your day to refresh and regroup. You'd come back from it thinking more clearly, being more focused and more attentive.

One of my favorite strategies for dealing with thinking symptoms is to take a break. In the same way that deep, restorative sleep allows you to organize your memories and "take out the trash" in your mind, even a short break during the daytime allows you to do the same.

I know, I know. You're thinking your day is already too busy, so how on earth could you fit in a ten-minute walk, much less a nap?

You may be right. Your day might be too full right now. But maybe you could think about ways to make some adjustments so that you can make the time. Here's a method to do that:

Step 1: Determine if you are worth making the time for. Think about your thinking and the brain fog. If it would help you think better, would it be worth doing? Is it worth your time to become more productive, fulfilled, and happy?

That's it. There's no Step 2. Step 1 is the whole method. *Decide you are worth it.* Then adjust accordingly. Whether you take a ten-minute walk or hide in a corner with a book (or even a coloring book), you'll feel better if you cut out something that's draining you and add in something that nourishes you.

Hey, you might find this a little flip or dismissive, and I'd agree, except for one thing. I've recommended this over and over to friends and clients, and every one of them who decided they were as valuable as the other seven billion people on the planet was able to find at least a few minutes in their day to simply breathe and relax. Sometimes it takes a little looking to find the hidden spot in your schedule to do that. But, when we look, we'll always find it.

Concentrate on Concentrating

One of the things that created the biggest challenge for me about menopause was switching from being a person who could pick up a task where I left off as soon as I returned to it. As a great multitasker when I worked with large computer systems, I might set two or three big tasks running, circle back to monitor them, and start the next piece when each one finished. It seems I never skipped a beat moving from task to task.

Ha! Not so any more. Especially when I'm writing. I'll work on a piece (like this section) and get two-thirds of the way through and the phone will ring or a pre-set alarm will tell me it's time for a meeting. If I haven't finished the section, I'm likely to come back to a half-finished

(Oops. See, it just happened.)

And because I have that multitasking habit from all those years, I *still* forget that I'm not good at it anymore. For me, then, concentrating on *concentrating on* the task at hand is a key component of accomplishing my day's work.

Fortunately, I've got a hack for that.

This may sound very "out there," but it's only putting together some pure science with some music. The hack has a name. It's called *brain entrainment binaural music*. Binaural beats are low volume frequencies that are played under the music, which is often soothing and non-intrusive (okay, it's usually very New Age music, but it doesn't have to be). When listening using headphones, we hear one frequency in one ear while another is played in the other ear. This encourages various types of brainwave activity by providing a brainwave pattern for the brain to "sync" to. Our brains naturally attempt this synchronization.

We have five different types of brain waves that are good for different types of tasks. They vibrate at different frequencies. During our awake periods, an EEG (which measures brain waves) would show a mix of all five types of brain waves, with various types taking the lead, depending on what we were doing.

Here's a rundown of the five types:

Gamma Waves. Gamma waves are the fastest frequency waves, in the 40-100 hertz (Hz) range. When they're in control and at optimal levels, they're great for learning and processing information. They're present during REM (dream-state) sleep. When they become overbearing, they can create anxiety or stress. If not enough gamma waves are present when you're awake, depression or inability to concentrate can be symptoms.

Beta Waves. Beta waves fall in the 12-40 Hz range. When our brains are operating primarily in the beta wave range, we're able to focus and perform logical reasoning tasks. Too much beta wave activity is associated with high arousal and stress, while too little is often an indicator of depression and an inability to stay on task.

Alpha Waves. These midrange waves (8-12 Hz) bridge the gap between conscious and sub-conscious brainwaves. They promote relaxed concentration, focus, and calming. Too little often results in gamma or, more often, beta waves becoming prominent, with a stressed or anxious feeling being the result. Too much alpha wave activity can create a drowsy or "day-dreamy" state, making us too relaxed to accomplish goals.

Theta Waves. Theta waves are slow and relaxed (4-8 Hz). They are present during sleep, especially restorative sleep, and also during deeply relaxed times. They promote connection with our emotions and with our creativity. They're good stuff, as long as they aren't over-present during times when we need to be more alert.

Delta Waves. The slowest waves (0-4 Hz) are delta waves, and they are associated with the deepest sleep. Many adults have difficulty reaching delta-wave sleep, but my dog and my grandson are very good at it. When delta waves are functioning optimally, you'll have deep, restorative sleep and a more powerful immune system, and you'll simply feel better. Hey, guess what? Menopause and delta sleep don't necessarily get along. (Yeah, I can tell you're surprised by that revelation.)

So, how does knowing all of this help you? You can learn what types of brain wave states help you. For example, I work really well on tasks like writing with alpha waves; I love meditating to theta waves; and, if all else fails, delta waves will put me out in a flash. I'll rarely try to sync to gamma or beta waves, because I get too hyped when I go there. I have bought several tracks of music and I use different beats or frequencies for each brainwave state I like to be in. They've helped me create habits. I only need to play the music that includes the brainwave state I want, and I'll start concentrating or relaxing or even sleeping.

As a special gift to you, I've created a collection of three ten-minute tracks (alpha, theta, and delta) for you to experiment with. You can get these tracks by going to menopause.guru/binaural.

Caution: binaural beat music is not for everyone. Please read the cautions included with your download and always try out a new binaural piece or a new wave type in a safe setting. If binaural beats don't work for you, a regular music playlist that you use every day as you work in a concentrated way may begin to serve the same purpose for you by creating a mental state associated with the playlist.

It's Not the End of the World

I told you about my "adorable foibles" way back in the Introduction—how, during pre-perimenopause, I would occasionally do the "walk through the door" thing, or mix up my work and my non-work calendars. (Yeah, I know you don't remember—that's why I'm reminding you. But only after I'd forgotten where it was—and I'm the one who wrote it!)

Well, here's the thing. We live in a busy, fast-moving, complex world. Information is coming at us at a pace it never has before. You and I somehow need to absorb it, catalog it, and integrate it into our lives, because we're supposed to be superwomen and do it all perfectly.

Or, wait. Maybe we aren't.

Maybe one of the basic lessons of this brain fog/memory lapse/ scattered brain thing is that we don't actually have to know it all, remember it all, and be the woman in the middle of the hub. We're going to talk about this some more soon, but before we get there, I want to suggest that one of your most important coping strategies is to cut yourself some slack. The world *will* go on if you don't buy the rice that's supposed to go with the chicken meal. Your children *will* survive if you don't make it to that one game. Your best friend *will* get over it if you're too distracted to notice that she got her hair cut.

Give yourself a break. Use your coping mechanisms, but don't worry if they fail. The world will go on.

Chapter Five

Can I Eat Myself Smart?

I admit it. I order the information in these books so that it makes sense to me. This is the way I want to see it. First, I described the symptoms that many women have, because I always want to know that what is going on with me could be described as typical, if not downright common.

Then we explored what's happening in our bodies that can cause those symptoms, because it reassures me to know the whys.

Then we talked about some "quick fixes" that can make life a little better, that can help us feel a little less out of control. Because control over my life is what I want, and I want you to feel like and to know that you have some control over your life now, even without waiting for the menopausal changes we're talking about to kick in.

In the next several chapters, we'll explore some of the things we can do that can make a long-term difference in the way we think, because

I want to be around for a while and it's important that I help my brain stay along for the ride.

In the next two chapters, we look at the first of my two favorite topics—nutrition and exercise (we'll look at exercise in Chapter Six). Right now, let's talk food. The way you eat really can make a real difference in the way you think!

How Nutrition and Diet Fit In

I personally believe that there's no problem, no symptom, no life crisis that the right nutrition (and the right exercise) doesn't help. This is especially true about the stuff going on in your brain right now. If you've been dealing with brain fog, "menopausal ADD," memory glitches, and/or the inability to multitask like you used to, supporting that beautiful brain of yours with the right lifestyle is more important than ever!

There are plenty of changes going on in your body that mean that your brain could be in danger if you don't treat it right. In fact, there's mounting evidence that some of the things that have traditionally been considered "psychological problems"—like depression and anxiety (which affect many women somewhere along their menopausal journey)—are connected to the health of our *gut biome*—the flora, fauna, and good bacteria that co-exist with us. Our biome's health is dependent on how we eat.

No, I'm not trying to scare you. I'm really not. But if you can protect your thinking, protect your brain, by making healthful lifestyle choices, why wouldn't you? Most of these choices are relatively easy, and they don't have to be in the form of iron-clad rules that you never break. Besides, most of them fit right in with helping us to keep our bodies fit and our weight at a place that feels right to us.

The Nutritional Building Blocks of Your Brain

You've heard it before: *You are what you eat.* Literally. Every day, cells within your body are nourished and replenished by the nutrients you take in. Every day, the waste products of cellular activity are cleansed from your system. Although your brain cells don't die and regenerate quite the way other cells in your body do, they do need daily nourishment in the form of the nutritional elements to stay healthy.

Here's a high-level look at the essentials your brain needs to stay healthy.

Water. Most of you is water, about 70 percent. But your brain is more watery than the rest of you—75 to 85 percent of your brain is water. Avoiding dehydration is critical for your brain function for lots of reasons.

When you're dehydrated, your brain shrinks and communication between brain cells, which is how your brain does its work, is impeded. Energy production is impaired and a vital component of hormone and neurotransmitter production is limited. The cleanup functions that remove toxins are dependent on adequate water. Basically, the symptoms of dehydration are brain fog, loss of concentration, and impaired short-term memory—exactly the symptoms we're trying to eliminate.

Do you want to make sure your brain has the water it needs? If so, take your weight in pounds and drink half that many ounces of water every day. Here's an example: If you weigh 140 pounds, aim to drink 70 ounces of water a day. The liquid that counts is water. Alcohol doesn't count at all. I generally suggest to my clients that they count ounces of soda, coffee, tea, and juice as half-ounces, due to the sugar, caffeine, and chemical content.

Fats. Fats make up 60 percent of the solids in your brain. No, I didn't call you a fathead. The fat in your brain isn't fat cells, like those in our bellies or hips, but sheathing that "coats" the glial cells that protect your neurons. Fat is also present in your brain in the form of cholesterol, used as a precursor for the production of neurotransmitters and hormones, as well as being a structural component of brain cells.

The fats that are most important to your brain from your diet are omega 3 fatty acids. These fats come from a variety of sources, especially wild-caught cold-water fish (e.g., salmon, mackerel, halibut), walnuts, flaxseed oil, and grass-fed meats. Although the cholesterol in your brain is synthesized in the brain, studies suggest that cholesterol-lowering statins may interfere with the levels of brain cholesterol, affecting thinking ability.

Proteins. Proteins are essential to the maintenance of the structure of all cells. Proteins are also essential components of brain hormones and neurotransmitters. These are critical components of the brain's communication system and are also critical for mood regulating systems.

Protein is also critical for every system and structure in your body. Don't skip it. If you are a vegan, make sure you understand how the combinations of vegetable proteins work to give you a full array of essential proteins (the ones your body can't make) and the building blocks for all 21 of the proteins your body needs.

Vitamins, minerals, and trace elements. Our foods provide us with vitamins, minerals, and other trace elements that are necessary, in varying quantities, for our health. These *micronutrients* are critical to our health. The interesting part is that we may not even have discovered all the elements that our bodies use and all the ways they use them. What we do know is that eating a wide variety of foods, especially fruits and vegetables, helps ensure that our bodies, especially our brains, have the nutrients they need.

Some of the micronutrients that are especially important in supporting healthy brain function are:

- *Folate, thiamine, niacin, and vitamin B-6.* Deficiencies in these B vitamins seem to correlate with confusion and memory loss. In addition, these vitamins together with the rest of the B-complex are critical to synthesizing energy from carbohydrates.
- *Vitamin C.* Vitamin C is necessary for the synthesis of some brain chemicals and for reducing oxidants (free radicals produced as waste from cellular processes) in the brain.
- *Vitamin D.* Vitamin D is actually a hormone, something your body can synthesize if it has the raw materials, which include exposure to sunlight. Vitamin D deficiencies have a strong correlation with increased risk of dementia. While I don't advocate giving up your sunblock, either spend a little time in the sun, sunblock-free, each week or take a good vitamin D supplement.
- *Magnesium.* Magnesium appears to block the brain from the toxic by-products of cell firing (or *thinking*, as it's usually called). It also has an all-over inflammation-reducing effect on the body, including reducing inflammation in the brain.
- *Zinc.* Zinc has recently been shown to be a critical component in the communication between neurons.
- *Selenium.* I mention selenium, in particular, because it is one of the newer health-promoting discoveries and is a micronutrient we are often deficient in. It's critical for the production of important antioxidant compounds. However, before you run right out and grab a bottle of supplements, know that it's possible to overdose on selenium. Only seek to supplement with selenium if you know your diet is low in this essential nutrient. I've seen 125 *micrograms* as a maximum recommended intake.

I've included that list not because it's complete (it isn't) but to show you that there is a wide range of nutrients that are required for normal brain functioning. The truth is that the less that food has been processed, the greater the chances of it retaining the nutrients needed to support your brain.

Energy Production and Your Brain

A few years ago, when I was still working in information technology, once in a while I'd have one of *those* days. A day when everything I did posed a challenge and I'd have to think it through and come up with a solution. Invariably, those were the days I was on the tightest deadlines, too. I'd go home ravenous, ready to eat anything in sight. Maybe with a massive headache, too, if I hadn't been hydrating well.

Because I was also in the beginnings of studying nutritional science and weight loss at that time, I'd get really confused by that reaction. After all, I reasoned, if your job was sedentary (and, let's face it, it's hard to get more sedentary than being a computer programmer), you would burn far fewer calories in a day than if you were, say, a construction worker. All the online calorie calculators show that.

So why did I feel so starved at the end of the day? Mostly, I would write those incidences off as "emotional eating."

Well, I was wrong. It turns out that, on average, the brain uses about 20 percent of our energy production just to do the normal day-to-day work of living. On an intensive processing day, that figure jumps significantly.

When your brain doesn't have enough fuel for energy, it slows down. It can't store infinite amounts of energy, so when it's used up what it had, it has to wait for the bloodstream to supply more. If your work includes a lot of brain processing, you need to make sure that your brain has the energy it needs.

What the brain uses for fuel. It turns out that the brain has a preference for blood sugar. It claims first dibs on any circulating blood sugar. And that blood sugar comes from eating carbohydrates. When it's not working off freely circulating blood sugar, it can turn to sugar stored in the form of glycogens in the *glial* cells of the brain. Glial cells are support cells to the neurons that perform all sorts of support services.

This preference for blood sugar and stored glycogen is one of the primary criticisms of low-carb diets. But those criticisms overlook one small detail. Your brain is just as happy working on ketones. Ketones are made in the liver from stored fat when there isn't enough circulating blood sugar to supply the energy you need.

Unfortunately, though, the body isn't necessarily efficient at extracting fat and producing ketones. During times when you are consuming relatively high amounts of simple carbs (sugars and starches), your body doesn't bother releasing enough ketones from fat storage to keep your brain happy until it's run out of blood sugar and stored glycogen.

What occurs next is hunger. Your body signals that it doesn't have enough sugar and starts to yell for more. Your brain gets sluggish because it doesn't have enough energy to work. You've probably experienced this. All you can think about is *food*. Your stomach is making angry noises. The new word for this is *hangry*—hungry-angry.

At the same time, your body starts to extract fat from its stored locations and process it into something your body can use. Fat is released as free fatty acids, which are happily devoured for energy by your muscles and most of your organs. Although this is a slower process than using available blood sugar, it will work for a long period of time (until about mile 21 in a marathon, say; that's when you "hit the wall"). Unfortunately, the brain doesn't work on free fatty acids. It requires those ketones, which are created in a separate process in the liver.

The effects of different diet patterns of brain energy. With the above information, you can begin to see what happens to our brains when we choose different dietary patterns. Let's look at a few of them in detail.

Low-carb or ketogenic dieting encourages your body to get good at releasing stored fat as free fatty acids and to convert them to the ketones your brain needs. It seems that this process is something that our bodies get better at with practice. The more we require our body to burn fat and produce ketones, the better we get at it.

What happens in the first few days of a ketogenic diet? After a day or two (depending on the activity levels of both brain and body), you run out of free-circulating blood sugar and stored glycogens. You probably don't get hungry, because the proteins you are consuming are slower to process and your body senses it has fuel. But your brain has a minimum amount of fuel to work with. It slows down and it gets hard to think. That's why a lot of people complain about brain fog for the first few days of a low-carb diet.

If you stick with it, though, your body starts getting better at pulling out the stored fat and converting the incoming fat into the ketones your brain needs to function. Your brain gets happy again and, if you're trying to lose weight, things are looking up.

It does need to be a sustained effort, though, because alternating periods of low carbs and high carbs creates confusion in the body. And confusion almost always results in storing more fat.

How about those intermittent fasting diets, then? What do they do to your brain? An intermittent fasting diet combines not eating for sustained periods of time, usually about 16 hours between the last meal of the day and the first meal the next day, although some forms use a 24- to 36-hour period once a week.

This encourages your body to release stored fat for energy in the morning hours. Many people find it beneficial and feel they are more clear-headed in the morning with this schedule, but there are a couple of caveats. The first is that if you find yourself feeling that *hangry* feeling, you're probably not doing your best work, because your brain doesn't have the fuel it needs. The second caveat is about cortisol. So far, we haven't touched much on cortisol (but look for a lot of info on it in the upcoming chapters on stress and sleep). If you get extremely hungry before you eat, you may be boosting the stress hormone cortisol. This can lead to fat storage, adrenal fatigue, and more brain fog. If cortisol is already an issue for you, this type of diet may not be your best choice.

What about those "lots of little meals" diets that were extremely popular a couple of years ago? These are dietary plans based on keeping your blood sugar stable all day. The theory is that eating large meals, especially if you're consuming simple carbs, raises your blood sugar (happy brain) and then, before your next meal, your blood sugar crashes (very unhappy brain). So, these diets ask you to space your meals out, eating small amounts every couple of hours.

Yes, this does work well for some people. It solves the problem of bottoming out your blood sugar and slowing your brain function. If you're one of those people who seem to need to snack or graze between meals to keep functioning, this may be a great strategy for you.

The bottom line. In truth, what works for you will not work for everybody. We each have different dietary and "brain food" needs. And we each have different lifestyles that make dietary choices very personal. When I work with a client around diet, I help her make the choices that are right for *her* life, not someone else's.

There are a few topics below to add before we leave the subject of nutrition.

Food Allergies and Sensitivities

At a luncheon the other day, I met a woman in her early 50s who, upon learning that I worked with women in menopause and nutrition, told me that she had recently been diagnosed with celiac disease, a genetically based autoimmune disorder. Someone with celiac disease cannot process gluten, a protein found in wheat and other grains. I'd love to say that it is rare for someone of her age to be diagnosed, but it isn't. Although it had manifested almost a decade before, the diagnosis had been missed until the symptoms became more and more pervasive and debilitating.

Food sensitivities, allergies, and even disorders like celiac disease can become more problematic and even develop as we go through menopause. Although the reason isn't completely understood, it seems that the fluctuations of our hormones create a greater sensitivity to our internal environment.

If brain fog is only one of a host of symptoms for you, it may be worth doing elimination testing to determine specifically what foods are affecting you. By eliminating foods from your diet for a period of seven to fourteen days, you may find that your symptoms begin to clear up. In general, you can either eliminate foods one at a time, or you can eliminate all of the suspected groups and then reintroduce them one at a time.

The eight most common food sensitivities are dairy (especially from cows), eggs, peanuts, soy, wheat, fish, crustaceans (shellfish), and tree nuts.

Alcohol

Do I really need to say that too much alcohol is bad for your brain? Okay. Too much alcohol is bad for your brain.

Am I saying you can never have alcohol? No. But alcohol is a poison that kills neurons in your brain when you have too much of it. That's why, of all "nutrients" that are ingested, your body works to convert alcohol to energy immediately. So, when you do drink, slow down. Allow your body to process it. Don't drink too much. And drink plenty of water, too, to prevent dehydration.

How Does Being Overweight Fit in the Picture?

Another question I get all the time when I'm talking about brain fog is whether being overweight contributes to the decline in our ability to think. To this question, I have to answer, "It's complicated."

I don't believe that obesity, in and of itself, increases the risk for mental decline or intensifies brain fog and other thinking symptoms in menopause.

But. But, often being overweight is correlated with other behaviors that can aggravate thinking symptoms. Often, we're overweight because we're making poor choices about our diets. We're spiking and then bottoming out with blood sugar. We're insulin-resistant. We're eating trans fats and too much sugar. And we're not getting enough exercise.

My answer, then, is that if you're carrying too much weight but eating the right foods and exercising regularly, you're probably not creating more risk for your brain.

Hey, Sweet Reader

Before we go on to talk about exercise, I want to let you know that I tried and tried to put everything pertinent for brain health during menopause years that has to do with nutrition and ways of eating into this section but couldn't figure out how to do that without making this chapter take over the whole book. So, instead, I put more information in a video course, which you can get for free at www.menopause.guru/science-of-eating-right. I hope you'll consider grabbing your copy, because it's got a ton of info about all the things we've been talking about here, plus more.

Chapter Six

Move More to Think Better

— • —

N ow that I've brought it up, let's talk some more about exercise. Everyone says that exercise is good for you, but how does it affect your brain and help you eliminate brain fog?

The exercise we're going to be talking about is not only about exercising your body, but also about workouts you can do with your mind. There's been ample evidence that both types of workouts make a difference to the ability to think and to avoid mental deterioration in the latter part of life.

Exercise Your Body

As you may know if you've read my earlier books, I love moving my body. I wasn't always that way. I wasn't a high school athlete. In fact, the one time I wanted to try out for a high school sport, I got sick and missed two weeks of pre-season practices, and cuts were over by the time

I was well. I guess I could tell you that that was the only reason I didn't make first string, but the truth is that I was well on my way to being cut even before I got sick.

Then, for years, although I raised an athlete (my son was a ski racer), I was rarely active myself. I'd promise myself I'd get in shape for ski season each year, but there was always something more fun to do, like reading or cooking or eating.

It wasn't until I was in my late 40s that I became a consistent exerciser. It wasn't even intentional that I became a runner. I was trying to lose weight, and my coach and my support group insisted that I had to be active enough to create more caloric deficit. They reminded me that if I didn't get and stay active, my metabolism would slow down to match my consumption and I'd stall out on weight loss.

What I hadn't expected were the side effects of exercise. Some were predictable—better fitting clothes, getting rid of my blood pressure medication, being in a better mood. But some weren't. I liked feeling better, and I fell in love with trying things. I became an adventurer. I became more confident and I met dozens of people who shared my new interests. At the time, I didn't care about the "brain benefits" of exercise.

Now I do, and I'll bet you do, too.

I want to tell you about four big reasons why exercise improves your brain health.

Increased Blood Flow and Oxygen

Exercise, especially aerobic exercise, increases your blood's ability to carry oxygen. In a previous section, we talked about the first two parts of the energy equation—water and something to burn (sugar or fat). Oxygen is the third part of the energy equation. Without oxygen, nothing burns and everything stops. Oxygen is required to burn fuel and create energy in every cell in the body, including our muscles, organs, brains, and everything else.

When you exercise, you increase the demand for energy burn in your muscles. If you haven't been exercising, the first time you tax your system, you'll notice that you're "out of breath." It's not that you aren't breathing; it's that the capacity of your cardiovascular system to deliver the oxygen your muscles need isn't there. You might also notice that your ability to think and communicate seems diminished until you "catch your breath."

As you continue to exercise over the next couple of weeks, you'll notice that it takes more and more exercise to create that out-of-breath feeling. Soon, you find yourself doubling and tripling what you could do before.

What's happened are three improvements. First, your blood has become a better medium for circulating oxygen. Regular exercise boosts the number of red blood cells, which are the oxygen carriers. It can also increase overall blood volume.

Second, your heart has become a better pump. Your heart, a muscle, is strengthened by cardiovascular exercise. It's pushing a greater amount of blood per beat throughout your body.

Third, more of your blood is being oxygenated. Our lungs have thousands of little tubes called *bronchioles*, where oxygen can be exchanged, but most of the time we use only about the top third of our lungs. Don't believe me? Try deliberately inflating all of your lungs. Think about sending air into every little bronchiole. I'll bet that unless you are a regular cardio exerciser, you actually feel a little discomfort as air enters some little-used bronchioles. When we breathe deeply while exercising, we start to open up those areas and have more of them to use for exchanging fresh oxygen for used carbon dioxide.

Reduced Insulin Resistance

Insulin resistance, as we talked about in Chapter Three, contributes to brain fog and other thinking symptoms, because it leads to unregulated blood sugar. Insulin "unlocks" muscle and liver cells to store sugar as glycogens in preparation for use. If the muscles are perpetually full of all the glycogen they need and there is still circulating blood sugar, when insulin looks to store the sugar, the cells don't respond and the sugar circulates until it is stored as adipose tissue (also known as *fat*—the ugly kind on your belly, hips, and thighs).

Exercise is one of the best ways to reduce or eliminate insulin resistance. As you use the stored sugar, the muscle cells start responding to the message of insulin to open up and store the sugar. It doesn't take very much consistent exercise for your cells to lose their resistance to insulin.

The effects of your improved insulin profile are better overall health and, certainly, better brain health.

The other way to reduce insulin resistance, by the way, is to wait until your doctor discovers it and puts you on medications that have nasty side effects. Isn't it better to do it yourself?

Reduced Risk for Heart Disease and Atherosclerosis

Two of the greatest health risks as we get older are heart disease and atherosclerosis, which is often called "hardening of the arteries." With this condition "plaque," sticky particles of cholesterol, begin to stick to the walls of the arteries, which are responsible for moving blood to all parts of your body. This narrows the pathways for blood flow and can cause pain in arms and legs, heart attacks, and stroke. In addition, the arteries themselves can become less flexible and stiffer over time.

Exercise reduces further build-up of plaque on the insides of blood vessels. This plaque comes primarily from the buildup of small-particle LDL cholesterol. It's this buildup that impedes circulation and leads to increased risk of heart disease and stroke. Exercise appears to help the body keep this plaque from building up in the arteries. That's because the circulating cholesterol and other fats are quickly taken up by muscle cells (including the heart) in order to fuel exercise. Of course, this requires that you aren't fueling your workouts by loads of sugary treats that simply replace the energy you've used.

There is some debate as to whether exercise can clear up plaque deposits that already exist in the arteries, but there is very little debate that beginning exercise, even when some deposits have already occurred, can help prevent further deposits. If you have been diagnosed with atherosclerosis, though, you should work with your doctor to begin exercising appropriately to provide the maximum benefit from your workouts. Walking is often the most recommended initial exercise.

Feeling in Control

Although this reason to exercise is not nearly as scientific as the first three benefits, exercise does help with feeling like you're doing something good for yourself. Unlike changing your diet, which often feels like pure drudgery until the changes start to show up on the scale and in your body, finding an exercise you love doing and doing it can give you an amazing feeling of accomplishment right away.

Just by going for a walk or riding your bike or taking an aerobic dance class, you'll start to feel like you've done something positive for yourself. Even if you have to start at the very beginning, you'll see changes very quickly, and they'll have an immediate effect on your health.

I've worked with many individuals who were very deconditioned. One woman had let things go to the point where she could barely leave her house and was forced to take long rests after walking only a few steps. We began working with 30-second intervals of activity and added a few seconds of workout each day. It wasn't long before she reported being able to go longer and longer between resting in her daily activities. Our first walk to the end of the block and back was a milestone never to be forgotten.

It's all about starting. And then it's about keeping going.

What's the Best Exercise for Reducing Brain Fog?

There are two answers to that question. The first answer is an objective one. Studies show that the best exercise to promote clearer thinking and reduce the risks of dementia, stroke, heart disease, and many other health conditions is dance. There's something about dancing, especially dancing with a pre-set pattern, that not only promotes good aerobic health, but also engages your brain and requires it to link to your body as you exercise. There may even be something in the connection with music,

This kind of dancing can include dance fitness classes, such as step, hip-hop, or Zumba, but it can also include "recreational" dancing, like swing, ballroom, or square dancing. The important elements seem to be that it engages your mind in remembering and performing the patterns. So, I guess figure skating would also count (it's too late for me for that one).

The second answer is that whatever aerobic exercise you will actually do is the best exercise for you for reducing brain fog. To get the benefits we're looking for, what you do has to increase your aerobic capacity. If you haven't been exercising, consider starting with walking, with at least some portion of your walk being at a pace hard enough to challenge your breathing. Once you're comfortable with walking at least a half an hour at a pace that's at least moderately challenging, you can consider whether you'd like to switch to another form of aerobic exercise.

If you liked the idea of dancing but are still in the beginner stages of moving your body, you can start by simply moving your body to music. Standing and swaying or even moving in your chair are great ways to have fun and get more active at the same time.

Anaerobic exercise (exercise that builds muscles, but doesn't challenge your cardiovascular system) has its place, too, but most of the known brain benefits come from aerobic exercise, meaning cardio.

Strive to exercise at least 30 minutes a day or about three and a half hours a week. Your brain will thank you.

Exercise Your Brain

While we're on the topic of exercise, what about all those sites popping up offering brain games, and the claims that playing them will help protect you from Alzheimer's and other forms of dementia? Is there anything to that? Should you be trying to exercise your brain? Will that help with menopausal brain symptoms?

Absolutely! Remember that old saw to "learn something new every day?" Well, "What did you learn today?" is not only a question to ask the kids when they come home from school. Our brains benefit from stimulation throughout our lives.

How Brain Exercise Lowers the Risk of Dementia

There are a lot of studies that show that staying active mentally lowers the risk of dementia. We benefit from both intellectual challenge and social interaction. Although it's not completely clear how those activities benefit the brain, there are some theories behind it.

Most theories about mental activities and dementia center around the concept that we learn things by creating connections between neurons. We remember things by using those connections and by adding connections between the things we already knew and the new things we learn. The more you use a connection, the stronger it becomes and the easier it is to retrieve that information. The more connections a piece of information has to other information, the easier it is to find that information.

Then, when something comes along that interferes with those connections, such as Alzheimer's or a stroke, there may be multiple connections between neurons that can form alternate pathways to the information you need, or the connections may be strong enough to withstand the damage. Or you may be able to develop new pathways more readily. Or the act of creating new neural pathways may inhibit the damaging agents in the first place.

Whatever the reason, it's clear that, although it may not be possible to prevent all cases of Alzheimer's or to fix all damage from a stroke, keeping the mind active is a key to minimizing the risks of losing your mental faculties as you age.

How Do Brain Exercises Reduce Brain Fog?

The thinking symptoms of menopause come from several sources, as we explored in Chapter Three. Some come from the hormonal fluctuations that stimulate an area of the brain one moment and go blank the next. The hormones that affect the way we think can be not only estrogen and progesterone, but many others as well. Other symptoms come from the changes in the way we think as estrogen stops the relentless stimulation of some brain areas, and we need to learn new ways of accessing those abilities. And still other changes come from a deep-seated need to understand ourselves in a new way.

How does doing a crossword puzzle or finding the duck flying the other way (one Luminosity.com game I remember from a free trial) help with that?

First of all, these games promote concentration. Most of the time, especially with the timed games, you have to pay close attention to win or to improve. If you're having trouble concentrating on tasks and you feel like you've forgotten how, or if you used to be a multitasker and are trying to learn to concentrate on one task until it's done, playing these kinds of games may help you develop the skills you need. If you find it easy to concentrate on these games and complete level after level but still can't complete the daily tasks of your job or of cleaning the house, consider whether the problem is with the intrinsic value of the task for you. Maybe cleaning the house isn't that important to you.

Playing word games can help if you're having problems recalling words and pulling out the correct word as a result of reduced estrogen in the verbal centers of your brain. These games can help reestablish and strengthen connections in those brain areas. Verbal skills definitely get better with use, so anything that encourages you to learn and use new words or use old words in new ways will help keep your verbal skills polished.

Even playing along with television trivia games, like *Jeopardy!* or *Are You Smarter Than a 5th Grader?* can be a fun way of exercising random memory skills. It also helps to watch how often the contestants forget the answer after they've buzzed in, too. You aren't the only one who "blanks out" when the pressure is on.

The important point of any of these games is to keep challenging yourself. If you can solve the crossword puzzle in pen without really thinking about it, or if you keep playing the same computer solitaire game over and over, you probably aren't developing or even protecting those skills very much. Find a new game to play or a harder version of the one you are playing. When I find myself applying the word "mindless" to my playing of a game, I know it's time to find a new challenge!

Does It Have to Be Games?

Maybe you don't like "playing games," whether it's the *New York Times* crossword puzzle or Minecraft (yes, playing the same computer games your teenager plays can help keep your mind sharp). Maybe you'd rather keep your skills sharp through writing or visual arts or even socializing. Terrific!

Just as your physical "workout" can be gardening or other productive physical chores, your brain exercise can be part of your normal day and not a specific workout. I find that when I'm deep in a writing project (like this book), I don't need or want to do a crossword puzzle or a word search game. I have enough opportunity to build my verbal skills just in trying to find the right word or trying to remember which vitamin has which benefit.

In fact, one of the most beneficial ways to exercise your brain is to learn a new "language." By that, I don't only mean spoken languages, like German or Chinese. You can learn the language of drawing—how to put pencil lines on paper to make it look like an actual thing (I'm super-impressed by anyone who can do that, because I can't). You can learn the language of music by learning to play an instrument or by joining a choral group. You could learn sign language. Or computer programming.

Exercise Your Passion

There's one more way, and perhaps it's the best way of all, to keep your brain sharp and to motivate yourself to stay healthy and fit for as long as possible. That's to follow your passion and make it a reality. Whether it's doing the job and career you've had and loved all your adult life, or whether you're ready to throw that yoke off to embrace a new passion, vocation, or calling, building a life around a passion can be healthy for your brain and body.

When I began my own weight-loss and fitness journey at the age of 48, I didn't realize where it would lead. Because of my own nature, I studied and figured out things about exercise and weight loss. I became passionate about it. I wanted to share what I'd figured out with other women. That's when I realized that it wasn't only about weight or fitness for me; it was about embracing the gift of menopause and living my passion, which is helping others find and live theirs, even in the middle of this craziness called menopause.

When I started living my own passion for understanding this subject and finding ways to share it, brain fog became a thing of the past. Verbal fluency? I rarely notice when I don't have it, because that only means I get to be more creative in finding ways to deal with it (like the ever-open

Thesaurus window as I write). Memorization? A little tricky, but worth the effort. Concentration? I definitely "do as I say" and use binaural beat music for improving my own concentration.

If you're already living your passion, great. Dig in deeper, expand it further; don't let it become routine. If you know your passion, but you've been putting off doing something about it, now is the time. I don't mean you have to quit your job and become a starving artist, but it's time to envision the path to living your passion and take some steps toward it. If you're not sure what your passion is, maybe it's time to begin an exploration; to find out what might really make your heart sing.

Chapter Seven
Ah, Blessed Sleep

—•—

*M*ost days were exhausting and Jenny was tired by 10 o'clock. But, by the time she'd finally finished her "chores," wiped down the counters, set up the coffee maker, and taken the dog out for his "night patrol," it seemed like her brain had turned back on and she was too wound up to go to sleep. She'd toss and turn for an hour or more, and if she did manage to go to sleep, she'd wake up as exhausted as when she'd gone to bed.

Jenny completed a symptom questionnaire I gave her and, based on her results, we implemented a plan that helped her get to sleep and sleep more soundly at night. At a session a few weeks later, she was excited to announce that, in addition to feeling better, she was finding that her job as a copywriter was much easier—she was retrieving the words she wanted and that wasn't nearly the struggle it had been when she hadn't been sleeping.

What happened to Jenny makes sense. Nothing makes more sense in terms of fixing your brain than sleeping well!

Remember baby brain? Back when you had a young baby in the house who was waking every two hours wanting to eat, wanting to fuss, wanting your attention? You'd drag yourself out of bed in the morning and by noon you'd be ready to nap with the baby (except, by week seven or twelve, when you were back at work, that was no longer possible). Remember trying to think during that time? I know, you don't remember anything from back then.

Well, lack of sleep is a hallmark of menopause for a lot of reasons. And that lack causes many of the same effects now as it did back then. Unlike when you had a newborn, fixing sleep is possible at this time of your life.

In this chapter, we're going to examine three issues about sleep:

- how sleeping affects your brain,
- how your changing hormones impact your sleep (like, why you can't), and
- what you can do to change your sleeping patterns.

How Sleep Affects Your Brain

Geek alert! Science stuff ahead.

Let me start with a fun fact about myself. I don't do horror films. The visuals are too intense for me, and I have a tendency to remember the images at odd times. I'm about to tell you of an online video I watched that I *don't* recommend to you (if you do like this stuff, you'll have to google it, because I'm not going to tell you where to find it, because I won't ever go looking for it again).

It was an old film taken of an experiment that occurred in the Soviet Union in the 1920s (I think) where the experimenters put about a dozen prisoners in a communal cell and deprived them of sleep over the course of about a month (no sleep whatsoever was allowed). By the end, most died, even though they had adequate food and water. The remainder were insane and skeletal, horrible caricatures of humans. That was one of the first confirmations that sleep is absolutely essential for humans.

For many years, no one really knew why sleep was so important or what its function really was. There was a lot of postulation that sleep was necessary for physical regeneration (and it is), but no one really knew how sleep affected our beautiful brains. Many thought that as we slept, the brain simply rested, except during the dream phases.

Recent research shows that there's a lot going on while we sleep, and all of it is important. That explains why, when we're not sleeping well, the brain-affecting symptoms of menopause seem so much worse.

Sleep is critical to forming memories that last. The original memory model that I learned in college told us we had two types of memories—short-term and long-term memory. Short-term memory covered the first few seconds or minutes of being exposed to information. Information we want to retain is transferred to long-term memory. Repetition of information ensured that the memory was stored permanently.

Now we know that it's more complex than that. Memory does, indeed, start with short-term storage. Then there's sort of an intermediate storage that allows us to remember the information for the next few hours. Then, during sleep the information is reorganized, connections are reinforced, and retrieval pathways are created. This reorganization is what actually allows you to retain memories long-term and to integrate them into your available information stores.

Memory storage seems to be associated with the REM, or rapid eye movement, type of sleep, which is also when dreaming occurs. It's thought that the weird and oddly constructed images of our dreams are part of creating permanent pathways to information that we acquire during the day. It is known that being deprived of REM sleep, which can happen with taking certain drugs, including the anti-anxiety benzodiazepines (like Ativan), interferes with the formation of long-term memories.

Another important function of sleep is that, while you sleep, the brain's glial and lymphatic systems scrub the toxins from your brain. It's thought that the relaxation of sleep allows the glial cells to shrink, creating more space between the neurons, allowing the maintenance systems—the lymphatic and glymphatic (so called because glial cells act like lymph fluid) systems—to remove the waste products of brain interactions, especially free radicals (oxidants) that accumulate during the day.

This process occurs especially during *delta sleep*, the deepest of the four stages of sleep. Delta sleep, when brain waves are at their slowest, is also the stage of sleep during which human growth hormone (HGH) is released at its highest levels. HGH is a key to restoring our bodies, healing wounds, and boosting our immune systems. There's also evidence that the presence of this hormone is helpful to memory as well.

Finally, although little research has examined or uncovered the reason, sleep reduces cortisol and stress levels. That connection is pretty well established. When cortisol is high when you're feeling lots of stress, sleep becomes problematic. But if you *can* sleep, you'll find that your stress levels are lower when you awaken. If you can keep yourself in a normal sleep pattern during periods of high stress, you may find yourself better able to cope with the stress without as many side effects. (I know, I know—easier said than done. Keep reading, though, because we'll talk about this more later.)

How Menopause Affects Sleep

Most of my clients have difficulty sleeping at some time during their menopausal journey. They aren't happy about it. At all.

Yes, the hormonal changes that happen in your body during menopause can disrupt your sleep. It's not only the changes in estrogen and progesterone that affect sleep; because those changes affect the levels of other hormones, there are lots of ways our sleep can be disrupted. That means that the insomnia that you felt during early perimenopause may not be the same insomnia you have once menopause has come and gone. I know: "Oh, joy."

Each hormonal imbalance brings with it a different pattern of sleep disruption. The good news is that this can help you figure out what is going on hormonally for you. In fact, this is one of the most important tools I use with my clients to help us figure out what's going on with them.

Here are nine scenarios of what you might be experiencing around sleeping and the hormonal changes they point to.

1. *I fall asleep fine, but wake up thinking (worrying, fretting) about all the possible bad things that could happen and then I can't fall back to sleep.* This is primarily an indicator of high cortisol. Stress has you thinking and worrying about what you're stressing about. Once cortisol is triggered, your body is primed for action, and so it becomes difficult to relax and return to sleep.

2. *I sleep okay (or I toss and turn and have a restless sleep), but I wake up "wired and tired"—ready to go, but still really tired.* This is another indication of high cortisol. You aren't getting good rest, but you're still ready to go when you wake up, because cortisol is driving you.

3. *I sleep plenty (maybe even too much for a normal person), but I'm really tired when I get out of bed. "Crashing fatigue" would be an accurate description of how I feel.* There are two possible causes of this one. One is low cortisol—what happens when your adrenal glands can't make enough cortisol to keep up. You just can't get going. The other is not enough thyroid hormone (or thyroid hormone resistance). Thyroid hormone is critical for

energy production and regulates your metabolism. If you don't have enough or your body isn't recognizing it, you'll get to this very low energy state.

4. *I wake up often at night due to night sweats (I'm so hot my hair's on fire!) or weird, vivid dreams.* Weird dreams and hot flashes are classic symptoms of low estrogen.

5. *I sleep okay, but I don't seem to have any stamina—as soon as I start a workout, I'm wiped out. A busy day is a killer.* This one is generally about low testosterone, which drops for some women in menopause. High cortisol or adrenal fatigue (low cortisol) can interfere with testosterone production, too.

6. *I just can't seem to fall asleep. I feel like I'm staying up later and later at night.* Having trouble falling asleep at night is often an indicator of low melatonin. That's connected with low progesterone. Melatonin supplementation can help.

7. *I go to sleep fine but wake up only a couple of hours later and I'm awake. I'm not really fretting, but I can't fall back to sleep.* If you're waking up not terribly worried or ready to go, but awake, this can be a sign of low estrogen.

8. *I sleep okay, but if I eat a sandwich or pasta for lunch, I crash in the afternoon. Same thing at dinner—I barely get the kitchen cleaned up before I'm in bed.* This indicates your blood sugar is too high, often due to insulin resistance. A walk before or after your meal can help, because using your muscles opens space for sugar storage.

9. *My sleep cycle seems turned around. I don't sleep well at night, but I could go to sleep in the morning and sleep all day.* This is another indicator of cortisol being out of balance. Melatonin puts you to sleep in the evening; cortisol wakes you up. Short-term supplementation with melatonin, while also working on

stress reduction and management, can help get your sleep back on track.

How to Fix Your Sleep

Rebalancing your hormones can be super helpful to fixing your sleep—and I've covered some of the ways to do that in my book *Lighten Up!*—but there are some simple fixes you can use to get in the habit of going to sleep more easily and getting back to sleep more reliably. Even so, realize that sometimes nothing works, and you might have a bad night.

Getting to Sleep More Easily

Create a conducive environment. Most "get to sleep" guides begin with telling you to create a bedroom that feels good for sleeping. That means it's dark, quiet, and free from lots of electronics. It's especially important to eliminate blue light, which keeps us awake. If you need a nightlight, it should be red or yellow light and as low as possible. They also tell you that bedrooms are for sleeping and for sex, but I've been reading in bed since I was four, so that's not going to change for me. If you find yourself reading until the wee hours, consider that changing what you're reading may help you get to sleep more easily. May I recommend a good statistics text book?

But those sleep guides rarely take into account the specific nature of menopause, and by that I mean hot flashes. If you're having night sweats, you'll want to make sure that your sheets are cotton or other natural fabrics, that you aren't "tucked in tight," so you can put a foot out if you need to, and that the room is cool enough. (If night sweats are really a problem for you, I've covered the topic extensively in my book *Chill Out!*)

Exercise early, not late. Just because your gym is open 24 hours a day doesn't mean that ten p.m. is your best time for a workout. Workouts *are* important, but if you're not sleeping well, it may be because you haven't left enough time for your body to wind down between your workout and sleeping. Think about scheduling high-energy workouts in the morning, noontime, or right after work. If you have to exercise later, consider completing your workout with a calming yoga or meditation segment to bring your body back down to a more normal level.

Make going to bed a ritual. One of the best ways to make getting to sleep easy is to create a routine and stick with it. Pick a time to begin getting ready for bed, figure out what *has* to be done before you begin your routine, and then design a calming preparation for bedtime. It could be as simple as doing a short meditation or having a prayer time. Or you might be a bath person, and a warm bath or even a warm shower could create a drowsy mood. You could then light a candle for a few minutes, read a short inspirational piece, or use an aromatherapy fragrance that's right for you. Whatever feels good to you, try it and stick with it for a couple of weeks. It might not work right away, but once that routine *feels* like a habit, it will probably become one, and that will help your sleep.

Listen to theta or delta wave music. In Chapter Four I talked about binaural beat music. Well, if you can fall asleep with headphones on, this can be really helpful to you. Theta waves induce easy relaxation, and delta waves promote deeper sleep. Delta wave sleep may potentially help you correct cortisol imbalances, so if doing this helps you get more restful sleep, so much the better.

Take supplements. If all else fails, there are sleep supplements that can get you over the short-term hump. I'm not big on using any of these permanently, but if you've fallen into a pattern and can't get out, here are some good choices to try that aren't drugs.

- **Magnesium** taken in the evening helps with relaxation (and sore muscles). If you enjoy an evening bath, putting Epsom salts into your bath allows you to absorb magnesium through your skin, relaxing muscles and helping you sleep.

- **Valerian and chamomile** are herbs, both of which are available as teas, which have long histories of use as sleep aids. The warmth of the tea can also help to increase the drowsy factor. (If you are on an SSRI antidepressant, there can be a dangerous interaction, so consult your prescribing physician before trying these herbs.)
- **Melatonin**, the sleep-inducing hormone, is available as a supplement and can be very helpful, especially when low progesterone is a factor. Tryptophan, an amino acid, is a precursor to melatonin and may be helpful.

Getting Back to Sleep

What happens if you get to sleep okay, but three or four hours later you're wide awake? I'm not sure there is much that's more frustrating than being wide awake when everyone else is asleep and you're going round and round thinking about what you have to do tomorrow (which, inevitably, can't be done in the middle of the night). However, yes, you can do something about being awake all night, waiting for morning to come.

Here are some things to try.

Intend to sleep. This is a simple method of making it easier to get back to sleep: You plan to go back to sleep. If you know that sometimes your sleep is being interrupted by the need to go to the bathroom, or to get rid of some covers, or even by a feeling of wakefulness, you may be able to simply tell yourself, "It's okay. I have three more hours to sleep, and I will enjoy them and be rested in the morning." By relaxing and perceiving your waking as normal, not an irritation, you may find that your next thought is when you wake up in the morning: "Oh, there goes the alarm clock." Even if doing this doesn't help at first, keeping this intention present makes all the other techniques work better.

Give up on worry. I know, you want to hit me for saying this. But worry is fixating on something you can't do anything about. Either you can't do anything, so you need to let it go, or you can't do anything *now*, in which case, you can forget about it until the time comes to do something about it. Yes, I know that makes sense, but I also know it's not so easy. I have a kid, after all. I know this.

So, if you tend to awaken worried about something that is going to happen, you can keep a pad of paper, a pencil, and a small flashlight next to your bed. When you wake up, write down what you don't want to forget, thank your brain for remembering, remind it that you've written it down so you won't forget it, and then go back to sleep. This works great for capturing those brilliant ideas you have in the middle of the night, too. If writing a note about it doesn't let you go back to sleep immediately, move on to the techniques below.

Practice gratitude. If I've woken with a truly fretting type of worry that's not about something I can do something about, I usually start with practicing gratitude. I list my blessings, especially around whatever I'm worried about. If it's about money, I'll think about all the wonderful clients I have and the people I'm helping. I'll feel the blessings of the material things I do have and of the abilities my husband and I have to generate income. I'll think of the thousands of ways we are rich beyond money. And I'll remember that someone else really is in charge anyway, and all I have to do is trust.

Breathe. My next best method is to do something called *4-7-8 breathing.* Popularized by Dr. Andrew S. Weil, this technique works well for relaxing at any time. When used in the middle of the night, many people find that if they do only a couple rounds of it, the next thing they know, it's morning.

Here's how it works. Breathe in for four counts. Hold for seven counts. Exhale for eight counts. I find that often when I do this, for the first round (breath) or two, I either have to count quicker or hold the breath for less than seven counts and exhale for less than eight. But by the time the third round comes, I have deepened and slowed my breath to the 4-7-8 pattern. I rarely remember the fourth round.

Progressive relaxation. I find this method particularly effective to use in the middle of the night. This is the one where you tense different muscle groups for five to ten seconds and then let them totally relax. Begin with your feet, then do legs, hands, arms, and then work up your torso—hips and butt, abs, back, shoulders, neck, and finally scalp. Try not to let your mind wander back to problems, but focus on what you are doing in your body. Don't worry about how far you actually get; I rarely make it past my legs.

Havening Touch. Havening Touch is a technique I discovered recently when I was troubled by a bout of obsessive thoughts. Havening touch is similar in some ways to techniques like tapping (EFT) and EMDR in that it breaks into the thought pattern and redirects it. However, it's extremely gentle, requires minimal training, and, best of all, can be done in your bed without disturbing your partner.

There are three elements to Havening. First, a gentle stroking, done by stroking the opposite upper arms with your hands, by stroking your face with your palms, or doing a "washing your hands" movement, stroking your palms together. This motion continues for the entire time (although you can switch between the three movements). The second element involves counting to 20 while imagining a repetitive movement happening with each count. This could be taking footsteps on a beach or path, walking down stairs, or even jumping rope. The final element involves eye movements done in between counts of 20. Without moving your head, look to the right and then to the left. You can do this with your eyes closed if you like. Do five sets of looking left then right with your eyes.

Alternate between the 20 count and eye movement three times (if you last that long). At the end take a deep cleansing breath. Generally, one round is all it takes.

One Last Suggestion about Sleep

If you aren't sleeping, but are lying in bed tossing and turning instead, because you can't fall asleep, don't do that. Instead, get out of bed, find a chair to snuggle up in and read a light novel or inspirational piece. Sip on some chamomile or valerian tea and relax. Usually, you'll find yourself back in bed and back to sleep in no time.

Chapter Eight
Stress Messes with Your Brain

—•—

When I saw my first meeting with Melanie come through on my online calendar, the first thing I noticed was that she'd scheduled for the first possible opening on my calendar. The second was her description of what was going on with her (a standard question I ask so that I can prepare for our time together). She described a growing problem with panic attacks, which she'd never experienced before. During our appointment, she described what had been happening.

The first occurrence happened when she was walking through the local mall. She found herself sitting on a bench, her heart racing. Her breathing was fast and shallow and she was looking around for a threat. She thought she was having a heart attack. Many trips to her doctor and many expensive tests later, her doctor told her it had been a "panic attack" and he prescribed Ativan, a benzodiazepine-class drug that reduces anxiety and helps with acute attacks, and an SSRI antidepressant.

Melanie happened to read my e-newsletter and remembered that I often spoke about how high cortisol and estrogen dominance can mimic anxiety, and she hoped I could help her before she became dependent on drugs. As we talked, she told me of what she affectionately termed "my crazy life." She didn't think her college-aged children with cellphones that made Mom too accessible or her parents beginning to make end-of-life decisions were the main cause of the anxiety, but her less-than-satisfying job and becoming increasingly disconnected from her spouse combined with the kids and the parents made her life feel "off the charts" stressful.

I wish I could say that over the course of a few weeks we removed all those stressors from Melanie's life, but you know that isn't always possible. What we did do, though, was remove the stress about stress and help her change what she could and manage what she couldn't change. Moreover, she no longer feared the occasional physical reminders of stress, the events her doctor termed "panic attacks." She realized that they simply signaled that her stress was getting high and so she'd give herself a "time-out" to de-stress. She never did fill those prescriptions.

Let me share with you the information that I shared with Melanie.

How Stress Messes with Your Brain

Cortisol, the hormone associated with anything more than momentary stress, is a big ol' bully. It's made in the adrenal glands and, because of its role both in waking us up every day and keeping us safe, the creation of cortisol is the number one task of your adrenal glands. If they perceive that you are under stress, they'll keep pumping out cortisol until they can't do it anymore.

The real "gotcha" in this is that if you aren't actually in physical danger or in a famine situation, your body's reaction to cortisol is to *feel* like you are in danger—heart pounding, shallow breathing, hyperaware. Sounds like Melanie's panic attack, right? Exactly!

But there's more. When your body perceives this kind of stress, it goes into reaction mode. "Reasoned" thinking, the functions of your pre-frontal and frontal cortexes, is way too slow if you're in danger. You need to fight or to flee *now*! So the areas of your brain designed for quick response, the amygdala and the limbic system, take over.

Thinking becomes less rational, and learning and long-term memory may be impaired. You become solely focused on what you perceive the danger to be and find it difficult to focus on anything else. Can you say "brain fog?" Right.

It's probable that stress and cortisol are more responsible for our thinking symptoms and for our feelings of anxiety during menopause than the changes in estrogen and progesterone.

But let's not completely count out the effects of menopause yet.

How Menopause Affects Cortisol and Stress

Women in their reproductive years appear to be less stressed, or maybe appear to handle stress better, than they do after the hormonal changes of menopause kick in. When you think back on it, it may seem like you had more stressors, with small children and a job and a husband (or an ex) and all that other stuff to think about, but it's not about how *much* stress you had; it's about how you handled it.

There are two reasons stress may have been easier to handle back then. The first is a neurotransmitter called oxytocin. It's been called *the cuddle hormone*, because a big shot of it is released when we're hugging or snuggling. It's the bonding agent between parents, especially moms and children, as well as a bonding agent between couples. When our relationships are new and our children are young, we're getting constant shots of oxytocin.

Oxytocin is the super-duper feel good hormone, much better than endorphins. When your brain gets enough of this one, you can deal with almost anything. As we age and as our relationships age, we seem to have fewer opportunities to cuddle and to get those big hits of oxytocin. Estrogen and progesterone promote the synthesis of oxytocin, so as they decline, our levels of this critical happy hormone decrease as well. This can become a vicious cycle, with the lowered levels keeping us from looking for opportunities to connect with our loved ones and fewer connections driving oxytocin levels even lower.

Then there's estrogen's effect on cortisol. It appears that estrogen modulates, or dampens, the effect of cortisol, allowing women to have a different response to an emergency situation. Some researchers have theorized and shown that women have a tend-and-befriend response to a threat, rather than the fight-or-flight response that is typical of men. In this response, women seek to get advice and help from others. It's a calmer, more thoughtful response and may indicate that estrogen is providing some relief to the amygdala and limbic areas of the brain from the stimulation of cortisol.

When we hit menopause and estrogen subsides, that modulation goes away. We may be experiencing cortisol in a whole new way, a way that feels like a panic attack or like a permanent blanket of anxiety. Frankly, feeling scared is scary. It makes us feel even *more* scared. What a chain reaction that becomes, because the more scared we are, the more cortisol we produce, so the more scared we feel.

There's another piece to the cortisol puzzle. Menopause, as an event, is stressful. The changes in our bodies produce a physical stress response as hormones fluctuate wildly. Those changes produce weird symptoms, too—symptoms we never expected and that we don't necessarily associate with menopause. So we stress out about that, too. Who wouldn't? We're accustomed to hearing about all kinds of dreaded diseases, and now we can't match our own symptoms to anything good.

What's the conclusion of all this? Menopause *is* stressful. *And* stress is bad for menopause. What can we do about it? Let's look at some solutions.

Some Ways to Stop Stress

What's to be done about all this stress? I wouldn't be so crazy as to suggest that you engage in "stress reduction." After all, most of the stressors in your life can't be made to just disappear. Even if they could, that would likely, somehow, create new stresses.

What I'd like to offer you are a few techniques I use with my clients to minimize the effects of stress on their lives and get back to thinking great and living even better.

Information

It may sound silly to say that information reduces stress, but doesn't it? For example, when I told you that our physical reactions to cortisol changes during menopause so that we feel more anxiety, wasn't that a relief? Doesn't it help to know that you're not becoming afraid of driving your car or washing the dishes, and it's just a cortisol overload?

Doesn't it make a difference if you know that the crawly-skin feeling you may sometimes have is most likely a symptom of menopause and not a sign of imminent skin cancer?

This type of information breaks into the cycle that gets set up between the physical feelings of our bodies and the sometimes irrational thoughts of our minds and allows us to simply... relax.

Mindfulness

Mindfulness can be thought of as "just being"—being present in the moment and with the activity or inactivity of the moment. When you go for a walk and use mindfulness, you concentrate on the actions and the feelings of walking and what you notice around you. You're not daydreaming about where you'd rather be or worrying about all the things you're not doing. You're not calculating the total of your bills this month or composing a long, angry response to a Facebook post you really shouldn't have read in the first place.

How does mindfulness help you reduce stress? First, it puts a pause in your churning thoughts. By allowing competing thoughts to slip away and only attending to *what is*, you stop worrying and planning. Second, mindfulness reduces activity in the amygdala, giving space to the more rational parts of your brain. Finally, mindfulness gives you a chance to regroup and decide what you want your response to a stressful situation to be.

There are a number of ways of practicing mindfulness, and you can start with as little as a few seconds of simply paying attention to your breathing or to the sensations in your feet and legs. Although it's probably close to impossible for most of us to spend a whole day mindfully, even spending as little as ten minutes mindfully will begin to reduce the stress load you're under.

Do you want to experience just a hint of mindfulness? Try this exercise (read it through first). Sit with your feet on the floor and your back unsupported by the chair back. Straighten your back. Close your eyes and breathe in a relaxed manner. Now, attend to every sensation that you can find. Take the time to notice each one. Feel your feet on the floor and the pressure of the chair against the backs of your legs. Feel your socks against the skin of your feet and ankles. Feel your muscles holding you up straight. What do you hear? What can you smell? How does the air feel against your exposed skin?

If other thoughts arise—thoughts not about what you are currently physically experiencing—simply thank them and let them go. If you notice that you've started thinking about something else, draw your attention back gently to a physical sensation you're having.

You could spend a long time doing this exercise and go deeper every time you tried it, but you can start with just a few minutes a day. Mindfulness can be applied anytime and in any place.

Meditation

Meditation is a time-honored method for de-stressing, but there are so many ways to meditate that you may find it more daunting than it needs to be. You may have even tried it in the past and given up because you thought you weren't doing it right. I'm not going to tell you the "one right way to meditate," because there are at least as many ways to meditate as there are people who meditate. When I went to find a definition of meditation that fit what I wanted to talk about here, I found many conflicting definitions that all claimed to be the one true definition of meditation.

I'm not going to embrace any single view of meditation for the purpose of stress management. But, to give us a place to start, I will simply define meditation as *any deliberate practice that allows the mind to relax and rest while remaining conscious (not asleep).* Mindfulness is a form of meditation—a practice of relaxing the mind and experiencing *what is.* There are many other forms of meditation that can help you take a break from whirling thoughts.

Before we talk about *how* to meditate, let's talk a little about why to meditate, what the benefits are for your brain. There are plenty. One source lists 76 benefits from over 3,000 studies that have been conducted on the benefits of meditation. I'll spare you the full list (you can see it at liveanddare.com/benefits-of-meditation) and summarize nine of the best benefits here.

1. Meditation appears to change the structure of the brain, increasing the density of areas associated with learning, compassion, regulating emotions, and self-awareness, while reducing density (activity) in areas associated with anxiety and stress.

2. Meditation enhances creativity and higher-level thought, in part due to increasing the ability to generate controlled brain

gamma waves, which are the most conducive to learning and highly creative endeavors.

3. Meditation improves focus and ability to attend to a task, even when the person has been diagnosed with ADHD.

4. Meditation specifically helps people make the choice *not* to multitask. In experiments, people trained in meditation switched tasks less often and completed tasks more frequently than those who hadn't been.

5. Meditation improves mental strength, resilience, and emotional intelligence.

6. Meditation enhances rapid memory recall.

7. Meditation promotes better relationships.

8. Meditation improves total physical health. The list of improved physical conditions is extensive and includes reducing the risks of heart disease, stroke, mitochondrial energy production, blood pressure, inflammatory disorders, fibromyalgia, and more.

9. Meditation reduces the stress response and cortisol.

If all that doesn't convince you to meditate, I don't know what will.

So, let's talk about how to meditate. I'm not going to try to convince you that you have to meditate in one way or another. I recommend a lot of different techniques for my clients, and even use different techniques myself.

Below is a selection of types of meditation that you might want to try. (Thanks to Giovanni Dienstmann of www.liveanddare.com for this breakdown. Please refer to his site for more specific meditation styles in each type.)

Guided Visualization. If you're new to meditation, guided visualizations are a great way to begin. Usually pre-recorded, these meditations allow you to relax into the words and descriptions of the guiding voice. The words allow you to create your own "mind pictures" to go with them and that helps to focus your thoughts on the visualization. Breathing techniques add to the experience and help you begin to train your mind to focus.

Contemplative Prayer. Practiced by many religions, including Christianity, contemplative prayer is meditation focused on a single word or concept that centers the meditation. In general, it is an attempt to open to messages from the divine.

Focused Attention. This type of meditation is similar to contemplative prayer, in that you attempt to keep your attention on a single object or focus for the period of the meditation. This could be a word or phrase (*mantra*), your breath, or an external object such as a mandala. As you begin to practice this type of meditation, it is common for attention to wander. When you notice this happening, gently pull your attention back to the object of focus. As you practice, you'll find yourself less and less distracted.

Open Monitoring. This is a method that uses mindfulness as meditation. You simply become the observer of your environment and allow your mind to rest in *what is*. A more advanced version of this type of meditation is allowing yourself to become the observer of your own thoughts. As you observe your environment, your body, and even your thoughts, the objective is to *simply observe*, without judgment—to experience *what is*.

Effortless presence. This isn't as much a type of meditation as the goal of most forms of meditation. This is the "quiet mind" state that many descriptions of meditation speak of and that extends beyond the specific time of doing a meditation exercise. For most of us, a process is required to get to this state. If you haven't been a meditator before, you might consider this to be a long-term goal, not where you start.

━●━

I have a few more notes about meditation to share. Many people can't sit still for meditation, especially as beginners. If this is you, any form of moving meditation might be a good choice. You can meditate while doing yoga, tai chi, walking, or even running. To meditate while moving, make sure you will be safe even if your mind wanders. Meditating while running in traffic is probably not a good idea. But walking or jogging on a running path can be conducive to a wonderfully mindful experience. Personally, I find swimming laps to be the most conducive exercise to moving meditation.

Then there's the question of listening to music while meditating. Music can be extremely helpful for a meditation practice. Those binaural beat tracks we talked about before are great backgrounds for meditation and can move you to a more relaxed state much more quickly than without the music. Some people find that simple, quiet music is very conducive for meditation. Others find that any time spent listening to music is meditative. Still others find that meditation is much easier for them without any music.

Massage

Massage and other ways we pamper ourselves aren't just silly self-indulgences or a waste of money. They are important tools for stress-management. Although the benefits of pampering are targeted for your body, they open you up to new ways of relating to yourself. When you take time for yourself, and when you allow others to take care of you, you get to relax into being someone of importance, someone who matters.

Massage promotes stress-management, because we hold stress in various parts of our bodies, and it can be difficult to even identify that, much less release it on our own. It's almost cliché to say we hold tension in our shoulders and necks, but many of us also hold stress in our foreheads, our low backs, and even in our buttocks.

Massage, along with hair and skin care, are also important ways of reconnecting with your body without being sexual. For some women (and I count myself among them), the changes of menopause leave us feeling unhappy with our bodies. I remember having gained some (more) weight and, one night, when my then-husband reached for me, I was too disgusted with myself to let him touch me. After that, I avoided sex and being naked in front of him. It wasn't *his* perception of me that made me do that; it was my own feelings about myself.

It wasn't until after we broke up (and I can't lie to you or myself—this issue was part of the reason) that I started reconnecting with my body. I started with exercising. While I was still in the "beat my body into submission" mindset of getting in shape, I was given a gift certificate for a massage, as one of those little "atta girl" bonuses from my job. I went in feeling a little skeptical and a whole lot nervous. What if the massage therapist judged my body? What if she laughed? What if I didn't like being touched?

I came out a convert. There was no judgment; there were no "shoulds" or "oughts." There was no "you need to lose weight" or "you need to gain muscle;" there was only acceptance. As for my nervousness, it went away because I felt in total control, even when I went to a place so drowsy that I couldn't have told her what I needed. I didn't need to tell her. My body was speaking for itself. It told her where my body was tight, hurting, or needing attention. My body had a wisdom that was unfiltered by conscious thought and that asked for what felt right for it.

The result of my "conversion" has been a commitment to getting regular massages and to caring for and listening to my body in other ways. As I've learned how to recognize the traces of stress and trauma in my own body, that's led to a lot of the deep-healing work I do with my clients.

It really is easier to think when your body is relaxed.

A Reminder about a Few Other Techniques

Throughout this book, I've talked about stress management techniques you can use at any time. Look back to Chapter Four to recall the relaxing effects of decluttering, building habits, and binaural beat music; and go back to Chapter Seven to recall the Havening Technique, progressive relaxation, and 4-7-8 breathing. And never underestimate the power of moving your body as a relaxation tool. These techniques, too, can remain staples of your stress management repertoire forever.

Chapter Nine
Can't My Doctor Fix This?

For centuries, wise women have treated their peers for the symptoms of menopause using a variety of herbal remedies. Many of these are highly effective for some, but not all, of the symptoms of menopause. As we've seen, the difference in diet, activity levels, and stress in earlier generations also probably made a good deal of difference in the way our ancestors experienced menopause, so that the symptoms they did experience were likely not as pronounced as we experience today.

And then, early in the last century, modern medicine took over and our options changed.

In 1929, scientists studying endocrinology (the science of hormones) discovered estrogen. They realized that women had drastically reduced levels of that hormone after menopause, and they reasoned that if they replaced the estrogen in the body, then menopause (and its symptoms) would go away. Hormone replacement therapy became a "thing" in the 1940s. That was the beginning of medical solutions for menopause, but it wouldn't be the last "instant fix" the medical and scientific community would try.

Later, doctors deemed that the "spare parts"—worn-out uterus and ovaries—were the root cause of the problem, and reasoned there was no need to keep these annoying bits hanging around after their usefulness was past. Hysterectomies (removal of the uterus) with bilateral oophorectomies (ovary removal) were prescribed for women, with increasing frequency, in the 1950s, 1960s, and 1970s. That practice has been largely abandoned, since it was discovered that there are trace hormones (estrogen and progesterone) produced by those organs that are highly beneficial to women throughout the remainder of their lives during and after menopause.

When neither of those fixes proved to be a panacea, doctors reasoned that, since the symptoms of menopause often mimicked depression, perhaps antidepressants—first Valium, then Prozac, and now a wide array of other drugs—were the answer.

But, as with most developments in modern medicine, as we continued to learn more, we found out that there were costs (side effects) associated with many medical solutions. Although I don't want to say that antidepressants are never the right option, I do want to point out the benefits and drawbacks of looking for a quick fix to thinking symptoms via medical, or even herbal, solutions.

In this chapter, I cover the most common medical and herbal options for menopausal relief, including why you might want to consider them and why you might want to avoid them. We'll look at them in historical order, starting with the oldest.

Herbal Supplements and Your Thinking

In culture after culture, you'll find that women have discerned which local plants and herbs are helpful and which are not for controlling the symptoms associated with being a woman. Herbs for cramps and heavy bleeding, herbs for pregnancy and childbirth, and herbs for menopause fill the *grimoires* of the wise women of every continent. It's nice to know we take care of our own.

Many of the herbs that are useful for menopause, though, aren't mentioned frequently as being helpful for thinking symptoms. That may be because they were not considered very effective for that symptom, or those who described or researched the effects of these herbs might have prioritized other, more iconic, symptoms of menopause (e.g., hot flashes).

Many of these herbs are phytoestrogens—plant-based estrogens— that mimic the way estrogen works in our bodies. Common phytoestrogens include black cohosh, red clover, and soy. Phytoestrogens carry the same risks for estrogen receptor positive (ER+) breast and endometrial cancer as synthetic or bioidentical hormone replacement therapy, and women for whom this is a consideration should not use these herbs or over-the-counter menopause remedies that contain them as an ingredient.

Other herbs that have proven beneficial for menopause include dong quai, maca root, kava kava, and evening primrose. For these herbs, too, there has been little direct study of their effects on brain fog and other ways menopause affects our thinking. Also, each has some possibility of side effects or there is evidence that they contribute to the risk of breast cancer.

I've covered what's known about these common herbs and their side effects and risks in an article on my website (and in my earlier book, *Chill Out!*, due to their generally positive effect on hot flashes). You can find the article at menopause.guru/misg/herbals. The herbs I've mentioned may provide you with some relief and, if you don't find yourself in a high-risk group for estrogen, you may want to try them yourself.

There are a few other herbs commonly used to promote clearer thinking and memory, and to reduce the risk of dementia, and they may be helpful to you in certain circumstances.

The two herbs most commonly mentioned in connection with memory and cognition improvement are gingko biloba and ginseng. Both have a long association with improved brain function. Gingko biloba boosts circulation in the brain and seems to protect against neuron damage. Ginseng's primary benefit is as an adaptogen, a natural stress and cortisol reducer.

Rosemary and sage, both common cooking herbs, are also considered beneficial for brain health. Both appear to boost memory and can be useful as essential oils or aromatherapy, in addition to use in cooking. (Essential oils can be used in massage oils or lotions, but generally should not be ingested.)

Other herbs that may be helpful include gotu kola (an Indian herb), periwinkle, rhodiola rosea, and bacopa.

In general, herbal solutions should be considered as medicines. While they can be extremely helpful in managing the symptoms of menopause, there can be interactions between herbs and pharmaceutical medicines, dosage issues, and side effects to be considered. When I work with my clients who would like to try herbals, I generally refer them to one of several good herbalists. Please be careful and do your own research if you choose not to consult a qualified herbalist.

Hormone Replacement Therapy and Your Thinking

Hormone replacement therapy (HRT) is a drug-based replacement of natural hormones, taken after the body is no longer producing them. There are a number of hormones that can be taken, but, in the context of menopause, there are two we most commonly talk about: estrogen and progesterone.

In the United States, HRT generally comes in two varieties—synthetic (pharmaceutical) and bioidentical. Synthetics are made from a variety of sources. The oldest and perhaps still most common is made from the urine of pregnant mares. Newer synthetics are made from plant sources that many bioidentical hormones are derived from.

The difference in synthetic and bioidentical hormones is that in synthetics, the chemical structure of the hormone has been altered in processing. There is no therapeutic value to this change (and it may make them less effective or potentially more dangerous), but it is required in order for the developing company to obtain a patent. There is a second, more subtle difference, as well. Although many prescribing physicians have become reasonably adept at writing prescriptions for synthetics so that insurance companies will cover them, bioidenticals are rarely covered and can be a good deal more expensive.

That said, let's look at two even more important issues: Are HRTs effective, and are they safe? Let's start with effectiveness. In a word, yes. Especially if you are perimenopausal or it has been less than six years since you reached menopause, estrogen can reverse or slow the processes that have changed the way you think. There is, however, a fair amount of research that shows that progesterone therapy undoes some of the benefits of HRT estrogen on thinking.

So, why not take estrogen? Well, that leads us to that other question: Are HRTs safe? There are fewer simple answers here. First, can you take estrogen for the brain benefits without taking progesterone? Yes, but *only if you have had a hysterectomy.* The evidence for this is clear. Estrogen therapy without progesterone dramatically increases your chances of endometrial cancer, if you still have your uterus. Moreover, progesterone has benefits that go far beyond the brain and into general well-being. If you take estrogen without progesterone, or in the wrong balance, you are liable to become estrogen dominant, which leads to another slew of unpleasant symptoms. If you are going to take HRT, you'll probably want to take both estrogen and progesterone.

Are there any good reasons *not* to take HRT? Yes. If you're at risk for estrogen receptor positive breast cancer, most doctors will not prescribe estrogen at all. In addition, studies on heart disease and stroke are inconclusive as to whether HRT provides a benefit or increases the risks. And there can be other side effects, like weight gain, breakthrough bleeding, breast tenderness, and bloating.

With these constraints in mind, most doctors follow the general practice of prescribing the lowest dose for the shortest amount of time for symptom relief. The average prescription runs three to five years. Many women have found that their "rebound symptoms" after stopping HRT have been much worse than the original symptoms the HRT was prescribed to address. This rebound occurs because the body seems to shut down its production of residual hormones in the ovaries, adrenal glands, and even fatty tissue when the HRT treatment begins. That production may never resume to optimal level.

There is one exception to this, however. Some doctors who primarily prescribe bioidentical hormones, especially those who are involved in the anti-aging movement, feel that it is appropriate to continue bioidenticals as long as the woman wishes to remain on them. The problem is that there have been few, if any, long-term studies done as to the effects of this type of HRT treatment. Therefore, the risks are largely unknown.

Let me sum up. HRT can be beneficial in managing not only the thinking symptoms we've talked about in this book, but many of the symptoms associated with the decline of estrogen and progesterone. But there are risks associated with changing your body's natural path through menopause. Ultimately, this is a decision for you and your doctor. I always recommend that women develop a good working relationship with their gynecologist or primary health care provider, so that they can discuss the right choices for them. Even if you decide that HRT is right for you, making the lifestyle changes recommended in earlier chapters will still be beneficial to your long-term brain health.

The Effect of Surgical or
Chemical Menopause on Your Thinking

Fortunately, the medical community rethought the idea that, after a woman has finished having children, her uterus and ovaries are no longer necessary and that a hysterectomy and double oophorectomy are valid treatments for a variety of medical conditions. Those conditions are now more likely to be treated with less drastic measures. However, there are still valid reasons that you and your doctor may want to consider those operations.

If both your uterus and your ovaries are removed, you are technically in menopause from that moment. The gradual reduction of hormone production that accompanies a natural menopause doesn't happen. Your body can be shocked by the sudden change, and menopause can be exceptionally difficult when caused by surgery. The instant change in the amount of estrogen may have an extremely negative effect on your thinking. You may find yourself with all of the thinking symptoms we've discussed, along with potentially dozens of other symptoms of low estrogen and low progesterone.

If you are in this situation, it's definitely worth talking with your doctor about hormone replacement therapy. A doctor with a good understanding of menopause can create a slow tapering into postmenopausal levels of estrogen and progesterone that would allow your body to adjust as if your menopause process was natural. In many cases, you can be prescribed HRT even before the surgery.

Chemical menopause is a term used to describe the deliberate cessation of estrogen through the use of drugs, generally Tamoxifen or Lupron, or as a side effect of chemotherapy. Chemical menopause is a common and important treatment for estrogen-receptor positive breast cancer and, often, for endometriosis. In the case of chemically-induced menopause, HRT is never an option, nor should you consider taking over-the-counter supplements or herbs that contain phytoestrogens.

A complicating factor for women dealing with chemical suppression of estrogen is that it may cause some version of *cyclic menopause,* by which I mean that, as part of chemical menopause treatment, estrogen is suppressed for some period of time. After that treatment, your period may return. You may return to menopause naturally or through further treatment.

If chemical treatment is your experience of menopause, it's critical to support your health through natural means—through diet, movement, stress management, and, most importantly, supporting yourself as a woman of strength.

Antidepressants and Your Thinking

Although HRT is prescribed to women in menopause to restore their estrogen and progesterone to something resembling pre-menopausal levels, doctors have other drugs in their arsenal that they may offer to help women cope with the symptoms of menopause. The majority of these drugs fall into two categories: antidepressants and seizure medications.

Antidepressants are often prescribed when the symptoms complained of are either emotional symptoms, like anxiety and depression, or the physical symptoms, like hot flashes. When an antidepressant is prescribed for depression or anxiety, it's because you may really need the help to get through your day and to feel normal or to be able to face the triggers for your anxiety. For some women, hot flashes and other physical symptoms are so overwhelming that normal life is almost impossible. If you're in one of those places with menopausal symptoms, antidepressants can be true life-savers.

The second class of drugs, seizure medications, are generally prescribed only when hot flashes are the major issue.

Although some of your symptoms may be taking over your life to the degree that you are ready to consider these drugs, if you are also experiencing the kinds of thinking symptoms we've been discussing, you may want to consider minimizing the use of these drugs. Because the flip side is that these drugs are the enemy of sharp, clear thinking.

The most common antidepressants currently prescribed for menopausal symptoms are SSRIs (selective serotonin reuptake inhibitors). Common drugs in this class are Prozac, Paxil, and Lexapro. A similar class are the SNRIs (serotonin-norepinephrine reuptake inhibitors), like Effexor and Cymbalta. These medications work on depression by keeping serotonin and norepinephrine—neurotransmitters that lift mood—in circulation longer.

However, those drugs appear to contribute to inflammation, which causes poor brain function. In addition, there is evidence that SSRIs cause cognitive decline, including confusion, memory lapses, and inability to focus. Those symptoms can all be exacerbated by antidepressants.

These drugs have powerful side effects and can be addictive, meaning that you may find it difficult to walk away from them, and you may require larger dosages to feel better.

In my opinion, just like with HRT, there's a time and place for using support drugs like antidepressants. When your life is really falling apart and you really aren't coping with the most important things in your life, then the choice is obvious: Get yourself back on track by means that may include taking medication, but make the lifestyle changes at the same time, so that you increase your chances of being able to stop using the medication. Although specific supports for anxiety and depression are beyond the scope of this book, many of the lifestyle changes described here will begin to support your body to move away from dependency on drugs to the freedom of being healthy and happy without them.

Does Your Doctor Have the Answer for You?

Menopause is a natural process that's part of the pattern of women's lives. Looking at a history of medical interventions in menopause will give you a hint that menopause has never been a particularly easy transition for most women. For centuries, we've looked for natural answers to the symptoms. Herbal remedies and, perhaps more importantly, community support for women in earlier times was crucial for getting through menopause.

As Western medicine matured, the medical community began looking for answers to what they perceived as a deficiency. Menopause was defined as a disease rather than simply a natural transformation of a woman's reproductive system to a new state. As everyone knows, a disease should have a cure, so medical science set out to "cure" menopause.

As the research community discovered, menopause isn't a disease. It's what our bodies are designed to do. Although it's not always a comfortable process, we can support our journey through menopause, rather than try to "cure" it. This is the stance I take with the women I work with.

If the natural lifestyle changes discussed in earlier chapters aren't working for you, or if your symptoms are so overwhelming that they're interfering with your ability to connect with your family or do your job, I encourage you to discuss the options in this chapter with your doctor.

Chapter Ten

Unwrapping the Gift:
From Brain Fog to Brain Shine

ay back in Chapter One, I told you that menopause (and even brain fog) is a gift. Then I spent eight chapters telling you why brain fog and other thinking symptoms happen and how to make your menopause journey better—how to cope and how to reduce thinking systems or make them go away. But I haven't mentioned the gift aspect for a while, like how and why to use the gift of menopause to enhance your life. What's up with that?

There's a method in my madness. Although I believe there's a gift, a magnificent opportunity, in the changes of menopause, I also believe that once you've opened yourself up to the messages of menopause, you don't have to continue to suffer with uncomfortable symptoms. You can feel physically, mentally, emotionally, and especially spiritually, fabulous. That's exactly what the change—menopause—is an opportunity to accomplish.

That change doesn't always come from knowing what's going on, who you are, and where you want to go. The physical changes are not only messages from your subconscious and from the memories (and often the trauma) that live in your body. They are often the outward manifestation of an inward process (one I will describe in this chapter), but they might also be the outward manifestation of a wrong diet, too much stress, not sleeping right, or not exercising right. Up until now, those symptoms are mostly what we've been focusing on.

Now it's time to understand the gifts that menopause and brain fog (or however your thinking symptoms are manifesting) have for you. It's time to look at these symptoms as signposts on your journey.

If you are tempted to skip this chapter, if you feel that fixing the outside is all you came here for, I ask you to trust me a bit longer. Everything we've done together up until now was only the beginning. Now, here in this chapter, is where (to use a cliché) the magic happens. This is where Madja takes over with her croning ceremony and Una becomes a wise woman. Hang with me here and see where it takes you.

The Mind-Body Connection

If you're like me, you always trusted your mind, your brain, a little (or a lot) more than you trusted your body. When I was young, I wanted to be a dancer, a swimmer, a horsewoman (that most of all). I had lots of ambitions that involved being very coordinated and fairly small. But my body wasn't fully at my command.

Okay, I confess, I was a klutz.

I may have been typical in that, but I was also raised in a household that valued the life of the mind more than that of the body. It was a world before soccer and softball became so universally available for girls. My extracurricular activities tended to be trips to the library and Girl Scouts and music lessons. My one foray into dance was disastrous, a two-week "taster" class while I was at summer camp. "Madame," an imperious-but-tiny Frenchwoman, told me in no uncertain terms that I had no talent for dancing. I was crushed.

As I got older, I became more convinced that I was not star-athlete material. Although I usually wasn't picked *last* for dodge ball, I was in that "negotiation" group—"Hey, you take Dulaney (my last name back then) and I'll take Stewart." The embarrassment wasn't much worse when I *was* the last one chosen.

I flunked the President's Test of Physical Fitness. Every year.

By the time I got to junior high, I soundly hated my body. I was confused by bras and periods and curves and a little too much fat. I wasn't cute, or pretty, or popular. But I was smart. I got great grades in my classes, I loved to read, and I loved to learn. So I became the teacher's pet, staying after class to discuss the reading assignment, or doing extra-credit work. I wasn't a total outcast, but I lived my life on the social fringes and inside my own head.

Even though I'd try now and then to master my body, it was always in the context of a fight. *Winning the war* on weight. *Forcing* my body to learn the skills of skiing or martial arts or kayaking. I was always learning to use my body with my mind, not my body. Even when I finally did learn the lessons that I've told you about in my previous books, the ones about loving my body and making peace with it and having adventures with it, I didn't realize until later that the issue was about more than mastering my body.

This relationship you have with your body is not only about loving this home you're in as long as you're alive. It's not even about your body being a part of you that you are responsible for and must care for. What it is about is your body and your mind and your heart and your spirit not being separate things. Your body *is* your brain *and* your heart. Your memories and your emotions live not only in your brain, but throughout your being, including your entire body.

Step Aside

For those of us who've always lived way more in our heads than in our bodies, this concept of being *all one* is scary. We've never trusted our bodies, but always trusted our brains, and now, as we deal with brain fog on our journey through menopause, we're feeling a bit (or more than a bit) betrayed by our brains.

I invite you to take a step to the side and look at this in a new way, from a different perspective.

A friend who is a brilliant artist and fabulous teacher is also a coach for creatives (that really means anybody who's willing to open up to their own creativity) who are stuck. She's the person who helped me formulate this next concept, although I think she and I visualize it differently

Imagine yourself on a road, your road. You're in a deep valley. You find yourself blocked, stymied by a gigantic pile of rocks in your path. You can't see ahead. Maybe you could climb over. Perhaps you see a small opening to one side of the pile, but it's one you'd have to squeeze through. Perhaps there's a path, or maybe more than one, that's a steep climb leading up a hill to one side, and there are other paths that lead into the deep forest (full of scary monsters).

In addition, there's fog, and you sure can't see ahead in this fog you're in.

But there's also a set of stairs, cut into the cliff on your right, leading to an overlook. If you climb those stairs and stand on the overlook they lead you to, you can look around see it all. You can look back at the entire road you've traveled. You can look down to where you are today, at the edge of a rock pile with the forest and the hills to either side. And you can also see beyond, to where each of those choices leads.

It's time to step aside and take a look around.

Standing on the Vantage Point

This vantage point, this place where you can see your whole road, is where I spend a lot of time with my clients. I invite you now to step up to this vantage point, to step out of the fog and look at the road, your road, that led you here; to look at your choices and your destination.

I invite you to see the whole picture of you: your past, your present, and your future.

At Peace with Your Past

The brilliance of the *pause* in *menopause* is that we have the opportunity during this change filled phase to recognize that we can stop and stand on the vantage point and look over our entire lives. We can see what we want to take with us as we go forward, what we want to keep as cherished memories, and what we want to let go of.

This time of our lives often includes intense experiences of letting go. Our children are growing up (or have moved out and moved on), our parents are growing older, and we recognize that they are moving on as well. Sometimes, we even see the relationships that have been the bedrocks of our adult lives coming to an end, as marriages fail to survive the test of time and careers fail to deliver on the promises that we believed when we began.

Recently, a favorite client posted a note that her youngest son had just announced he no longer believed in Santa Claus. That milestone, while from the outside was such a small thing, was a marker for her of the beginning of the end of the time during which she could safely rely on knowing her role in life. For her, that also marked the beginning of a time of taking on new roles she's discovered and is passionate about. And so, for her, it's a time of sadness, but also one of anticipation.

When I reached that point, I let go of all four of those former bedrocks: My son grew up and started to live his own life; my marriage fell apart; I helped my mother move on from this life to whatever comes next; and I began to see my career in information technology as too small to hold my dreams. Over the course of the six or so years of perimenopause, I let go of so much.

When we are standing on the vantage point, we also learn something else. We look at the chokepoint in the road, that pile of rocks, with the hills on one side, the forest on the other, and, if we care to look, we see that we've been carrying a burden, a giant sack of "stuff" we've picked up all along our road.

That sack of stuff is getting in the way of moving forward. It's too big to fit between the trees, too heavy to carry over the rocks, too bulky to drag up the hills. There's nothing worth saving in there anyway, because, if you look back, you can see that you've been dragging along a sack filled with the worst, filled with the baggage of all the traumas you've ever had.

Make peace with your past. This is a big gift of menopause, of your vantage point.

This isn't about therapy. There's a lot to be said for therapy, and many of my clients have done magnificent work in therapy. I have, myself. Therapy is often about *processing* trauma. (Trauma is defined as any event that is too much to process in the moment. We've all had traumas, big and small, in our lives, and for most of us, we haven't gone back to process them.)

The work we do in life coaching is different. It is about recognizing the way the past is affecting your decisions today and changing the way you move forward. It's about knowing that you'll be affected by the process and choosing, in the moment, to act differently, to try something new. It's about recognizing the lies you believe about yourself and the world—doing that in order to get past the trauma—and deciding not to believe them. It's about acknowledging how strong and resilient you were and are to have survived that trauma and made it this far.

You look in your sack and you throw out a lie, a burden. Maybe you crack a rock that looks like a lie, and in the center is a diamond or a ruby—a brilliant gem of a memory of how you survived and maybe even thrived, or the shimmer of a life lesson learned that you'll always remember. As you let go of the stuff that doesn't work, that didn't work, you turn those heavy rocks into gems of memories of wonderful moments. You *magic* the rocks in your sack into a little pouch of gemstones.

Unfortunately, this process is about making that decision to turn the rocks of your life into gemstones over and over. Because, just when you think everything is a-okay, something happens in your life and you find that rock that you threw out. It's right back in the sack, a lump of hardness surrounding the gem you thought you'd polished. But it's smaller this time. You can recognize the lie, the burden, again, and toss it out. Again.

It's not the lie itself that separates you from your life. It's *believing* the lie.

It's so much easier to carry that little pouch of gems than the burdens of the past, isn't it?

Engaged in Your Present

The present is all about that chokepoint, that block in the road that you find yourself up against. But is it really a chokepoint? Is it really keeping you from moving forward? Or is it just pointing out to you the choices you have?

Many of my clients come to me identifying "menopause" (or one of its symptoms) as the pile of rocks in their road, as the thing they can't get past. They're so absorbed in looking at the rocks that they're not even recognizing the path on the hill or the one through the forest. They see the rock pile as huge, insurmountable, and imagine that it goes on forever.

They don't see that it's also strewn with magnificent gems, lying there for them to pick up, examine, and discover. When they step to the vantage point, they can see it all. They see the gems in the rock pile. They can even see that if they break up some of those rocks, they'll find even more gems. They see that the monsters in the forest are chained so they can't reach the path. They see that the path up the hill, once they've squeezed through that gap with their smaller sack, actually goes along a very gentle slope.

Yes, there's work to be done. There's no denying it. But from here, this vantage point, you can see that the work isn't impossible, and the way forward isn't blocked. Most of all, you can see that, on the other side, there's something worthwhile. There's a bright future.

Excited About Your Future

Perhaps the best thing of all about this vantage point is that from it, you can see what lies ahead, your future. Oh, you have a future all right. And it's not the same as your past. This is one of the things I hope you've learned from all this discussion about how your brain changes. You aren't the same person you were. But, then again, you weren't the same person after you went to college or met your husband or had your babies, were you?

So, *how* do you make this change of looking to your future? What is this new you going to look like? How will you fit into the world?

From the vantage point, you can see choices. Look around. What paths and options do you notice? Do they all lead to the same place for you? If so, does that make your heart sing? Or do you see multiple destination options for your life that you want to explore?

You get to choose where you go from here.

The deepest secret of all is that those destinations aren't "out there" somewhere. Whatever you want your life to be, you get to choose it, but you also get to create it. You get to have magic in your life. This is not just happening to you, it's happening through you.

You, Reimagined

You get to create your future. You get to decide who you want to be in it. You get to stand on this vantage point and imagine what you want in your future and then decide to be that person. It may not always be easy to be that new person. If you're like me, you'll slip back into being the old you, the scared or frustrated or tired-and-can't-go-on you, more times than you'd like to admit.

But knowing that this vantage point—the one from which you can always see the future you want to have—is inside you, *always*, means you can always go there. If you lose the vision, simply step back to it. The more often you step up to that vantage point to see where you're headed, the easier it gets to reach it.

Your own vantage point can't be reached just by using your mind, your brain. You get there by including all of yourself—your mind, your heart, your spirit, and your body.

Earlier this week, as I was writing this chapter to explain what my heart knows and what my body knows, I was struggling. The words weren't coming. I would open the document on my computer and stare at the blank screen. I'd write a few words and then I'd delete them.

Then I went for a run. I had a misstep, stepping badly on the edge between road and shoulder; I almost fell and I twisted my ankle. No lasting damage was done, fortunately, but it was a sharp (and very painful) reminder not to lose touch with my body. The next day, I danced. I did a long, complicated, sweaty dance, during which my head and my body and my emotions and my spirit all worked together in joy and in peace.

This morning, I knew what to write, because I had reconnected with all of myself.

You take all of yourself on this journey. And you choose what parts of yourself you want to take forward.

——•——

My client Anne had an epiphany. She came to me because she didn't understand what was happening in her mind. She was confused by the changes in her body, and just plain confused—she felt foggy and "off" most of the time. She was scared and angry, because she treasured her ability to think and it was deserting her.

Together, we examined all the things we've talked about here. Anne was fascinated, like most of my clients are, with the science. She was diligent with her diet and excited about her exercise. Her sleep became deeply restorative.

But she resisted opening the gift of shifted perspective. She veered away from stepping up to the vantage point. Instead, she returned to the rock pile. She didn't want to take the next step.

She felt better. She returned to work each Monday with renewed vigor. And it had only taken a couple of weeks to get her there.

But.

But she still felt *off*. Other symptoms began cropping up. She wanted it all to stop, so she could just feel like herself again. Finally, frustration won out and she agreed to examine what was really going on.

In a session where we began the deep work we, symbolically, climbed to the vantage point. I asked her to find the markers of the past in her body and look for the lessons her body had for her. She did, and then she looked to her future and began to create a vision of where she wanted to go. She also saw herself clearly in the present.

She had work to do. She had gems to mine and polish. But her path was clear, and she had a steady vision to keep her going. Upon the completion of our work together Anne said, "I'm at peace with my past, engaged in my present, and excited about my future."

The last time I talked to her, which was a few weeks ago, she'd planned her exit strategy from a job she knew wouldn't fulfill her deepest desires, and she was moving forward with her artwork, creating the future she saw from her vantage point.

Chapter Eleven

Me and You

Dearest Reader,

Now that we've spent these pages together and know each other a little better, I'd like to share with you a bit more about my journey. I started all this research and this menopause writing and coaching, because I needed it. For me, in perimenopause I felt like I was being ejected from my own life. I was depressed and overweight, but more than that, I had lost my shine. I felt like the mostly outsider I had been in high school. Again.

I just wanted to feel like myself again. The me who belonged. The me who thought she liked herself.

My own journey through menopause started with the life hacks, the diet, and a focus on the physical changes. I thought that would be enough to get me though and, honestly, it felt great to feel great. When I work with women who "just want to lose weight" (and I help plenty of women who start out that way), they do feel fantastic when the weight starts dropping and their clothes start fitting better.

I mostly write about that part of the journey—about the science stuff that underlies what's changing in your body and your life, and how you can minimize the madness of your life. That's the reason the majority of this book is about the science and the hacks and the fixes.

There are a couple of reasons that I do it this way.

The first is simply that I love science. I really do. I love understanding what's going on, and I love explaining it in a way that someone who doesn't have the time to go digging through the journals and the Internet can understand it. I love looking at opposing viewpoints and fact-checking the evidence. I love the insights that doing all that gives me.

The second reason I've presented things the way I have is that you need that information. Even if it's only reading through it once and then forgetting everything you read. Because once you know that there's something rational behind what's happening to you, once you understand that there's still logic (and science) operating, you realize that you can take back some control. You can make a difference in the way you experience your life.

And, finally, I do it because you probably need some help fixing your body. I'll bet that, for you, one or more symptoms of menopause has become pretty darn annoying. Maybe even debilitating. Even if that symptom is a message, I'll bet you'd be happier if it went away. That requires supporting your body, mind, heart, and spirit with real, physical, tangible actions.

When a woman comes to me for coaching, it's usually around wanting to change her real, physical, tangible symptoms. But then we go deeper. We look at the symptoms and what they might mean. We decode the messages. We unwrap the gifts.

I'd like you to meet Lena. Lena came to me first about weight loss. But when we talked for the first time, she told me she was miserable. The weight gain was only the most obvious and annoying symptom. She had others, including brain fog, but mostly she didn't love her life anymore.

She had a job, but it was only a job. Years ago, she'd thought it might be something she'd love, but it had turned into only a job. She was good at it, but it wasn't enough. She was caught in a marriage she was ambivalent about but she still had teenagers at home and wasn't ready to chuck the marriage. Her life was comfortable, but it wasn't fulfilling.

When we started working together, we first fixed her diet. We worked on helping her stick with it, and on getting back to it when she'd strayed. We busted through a couple of plateaus. We made some changes to other physical things that weren't working. We even dealt with her cortisol issues. We addressed the stuff I cover in *Lighten Up!*, and that I cover in the middle chapters of this book.

As important as all of that was, it was preliminary. I wish you could see Lena shining now! She went to her vantage point and looked around. She dug into her past and let go of old patterns and stopped telling herself lies she'd believed since childhood. She found new passion for her job and for her marriage. Even so, she decided to leave her job. She devised an exit strategy for her job and decided that, for her, it was worth recommitting to her marriage. She created a vision for her future and began actively pursuing its creation. She and her husband are planning a "second honeymoon" getaway and are redesigning their life together.

That's what menopause is all about. Getting through menopause is not about weight loss or managing hot flashes, or even thinking again. It's about you, reimagined.

Because the gift of menopause is *you*.

Jeanne

Further Reading from the Menopause Guru

- *I Just Want to Be ME Again!: A Guide to Thriving through Menopause*
- *Lighten Up!: A Game Plan for Losing Weight for Women in Menopause*
- *Chill Out!: A Natural Approach for Controlling Hot Flashes*

Acknowledgments

In any heroine's journey, no matter what the quest, there will be those who stand with lanterns to point the way, those who invite the heroine into their homes for rest and refreshment. There will be wise women with cryptic advice (always useful at junctures the wise woman foresaw, but the heroine didn't). There will be brave fellow adventurers. There will even be apprentice heroines who eventually prove to be more adept than the seasoned heroine. And there will be those who celebrate the triumphant return of the heroine, with great rejoicing, while celebrating their own triumphs as well.

We are all heroines. Every one of us. We embarked on the voyage of life and we have the opportunity to choose to take center stage in our own lives. The more I write, the more I embrace this heroine's journey. Although I am not the boldest and bravest heroine out there, I still like to think of my own journey as being heroic.

I would like to acknowledge some of the heroines who have helped me in my journey of this book.

First and foremost, I would like to thank Hillary Rodham Clinton and her magnificent sidekicks, Michelle Obama and Elizabeth Warren, for modeling that a true heroine always aims high. This book is dedicated to them, in gratitude for their personal sacrifice, for their never-ending grace, and for showing us that menopausal women *do* have a place in our world.

To my sometimes workmate/playmate and always friend, Nikki Jackson, thank you for our work sessions. They keep me honest.

I thank my publisher, Difference Press; its leader, Angela Lauria Kingdom; and its magnificent majordomo, Paul Brycock Kingdom. Thank you both for being so much: the wise woman with cryptic advice, the lantern-bearer pointing the way, the welcoming hearth for rest and refreshment on my journey. And thanks to my editor, Grace Kerina, who always makes me sound better than I write. Thanks, always, beautiful ones!

To the Morgan James Publishing team: Special thanks to David Hancock, CEO & Founder for believing in me and my message. To my Author Relations Manager, Margo Toulouse, thanks for making the process seamless and easy. Many more thanks to everyone else, but especially Jim Howard, Bethany Marshall, and Nickcole Watkins.

Thanks also to my sidekicks—the members of The Order of the Plume and the members of The Mystic Krewe of Nyx. Every one of you is a heroine in my story and in yours.

We ride!

About the Author

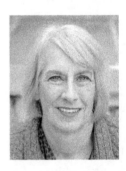 Jeanne Andrus is a woman with a passion for helping women come through their menopausal journeys with renewed health and an excitement for life that they may have thought was gone forever.

After years of neglecting herself while pursuing motherhood and a corporate career, at the age of 48, Jeanne committed to health and self-fulfillment in the wake of her divorce. Her new-found love for fitness and health helped her lose 80 pounds, renew her passion for outdoor adventure, and create the life of her dreams.

That dream included creating a business as a certified personal trainer and health coach (certified by the American Council on Exercise). Coaching women for fitness and weight loss led Jeanne to realize how pervasive the changes of perimenopause and menopause are and led her to create a holistic coaching approach to midlife and weight loss that she calls Menopause Mastery Coaching.

Recently, she has incorporated her reiki practice into her coaching, offering healing sessions that examine the underlying emotional and physical issues influencing the symptoms women experience during perimenopause and menopause.

When she's not coaching her worldwide clients from her home in the Greater New Orleans area, she's off adventuring—doing anything from visiting her grandson and skiing in New England to scuba diving in Belize.

Website: www.menopause.guru and www.menopausebooks.com.
Email: jeanne@menopause.guru
Facebook: www.facebook.com/menopauseguru

Thank You

Without your interest in the topic of menopause, writing this book would have been a much more boring task. I want to express my appreciation for you for taking the time to explore becoming the best you you've ever been. If that wasn't your goal, you wouldn't still be reading.

Most of you are busy women with lots on your plates (figuratively or literally) and who don't have time do the research it takes to know how to support you bodies, but you're still intensely interested in the topic of menopause and how it relates to you.

I've created something special for you, my reader: *The Science of Eating Right for Menopause*, a five-part video course (with notes and transcripts) of additional information I couldn't fit in this book. It's the information I give my one-on-one clients when they're confused about how to eat right and why their diet isn't working.

You can get access to this course right now at www.menopause.guru/science-of-eating-right. I hope you enjoy it as much as I enjoyed creating it for you.

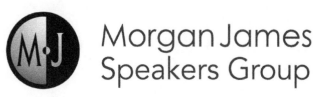

Morgan James
Speakers Group

We connect Morgan James published
authors with live and online events
and audiences whom will benefit
from their expertise.

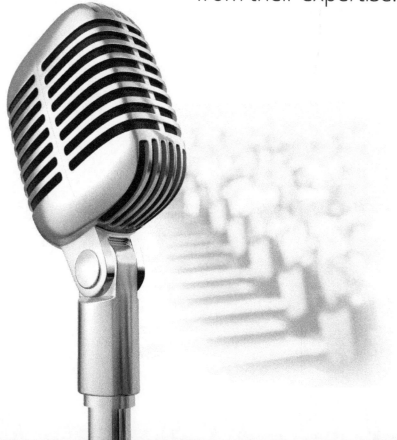

Morgan James makes all of our titles available
through the Library for All Charity Organization.

www.LibraryForAll.org

Printed in the USA
CPSIA information can be obtained
at www.ICGtesting.com
JSHW082356140824
68134JS00020B/2105